COLOUR G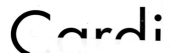

Cardi

Mc
Car

Pe
Con

Ar
Briti
Hor

SE

EDINBURGH LONDON NEW YORK PHILADELPHIA SYDNEY
TORONTO 1997

CHURCHILL LIVINGSTONE
A Medical Division of Harcourt Brace and Company Limited

© Longman Group UK Ltd 1993
© Pearson Professional Limited 1997
© Harcourt Brace and Company Limited 1999

🕭 is a registered trademark of Harcourt Brace and Company Limited

M. Lowe, P. Schofield and A. Grace have asserted their right under the Copyright, Designs and Patents Act, 1988, to be identified as Authors of this work.

First published as Colour Guide Cardiology 1993
Second edition 1997
   Reprinted 1998

ISBN 0 443 059128

British Library Cataloguing in Publication Data
A catalogue record for this book is available from the British Library.

Library of Congress in Publication Data
A catalog record for this book is available from the Library of Congress.

Medical knowledge is constantly changing. As new information becomes available, changes in treatment, procedures, equipment and the use of drugs become necessary. The editors/authors/contributors and the publishers have, as far as it is possible, taken care to ensure that the information given in this text is accurate and up to date. However, readers are strongly advised to confirm that the information, especially with regard to drug usage, complies with current legislation and standards of practice.

The publisher's policy is to use **paper manufactured from sustainable forests**

For Churchill Livingstone

Publisher: Laurence Hunter
Project Editor: James Dale
Production: Kay Hunston
Design direction: Erik Bigland

Printed in China
SWTC/02

Preface

Technical advances in cardiology occur at an astonishing rate but should not obscure the principal objectives of physicians, namely alleviating suffering and improving the outlook of our patients. Despite a necessary but increasing emphasis on modern technology, well established tenets, including the history and physical examination, remain cornerstones that should guide practice. The purpose of this book continues to be to give a broad, and we hope balanced, overview of modern practice both for those approaching this branch of medicine for the first time and for those who regularly contribute to the management of patients with cardiovascular disease.

In the task of collecting images for the book we have received invaluable help, as previously, from many colleagues. Four individuals in particular deserve our special thanks: Dr Jim Hall, a co-author for the first edition has been, as usual, generous in his support; Dr Hugh Fleming, Senior Consultant Cardiologist, Papworth Hospital, 1959–1988, deserves our sincere thanks for allowing us to use photographs, many of which were taken by himself, and that were used extensively in his clinical teaching (Figures 1, 8, 27, 46, 58–9, 83–4, 89, 93–4, 107–8, 112, 114, 119, 158–9, 165, 169–70, 172, 176, 182–3, 189, 194); Dr Nat Cary for supplying many of the pathological images and his critical comments on the text; and Professor Bob Anderson of the National Heart and Lung Institute for his much appreciated criticism and the striking images of complex congenital anomalies (Figs 171, 180). Our colleagues and friends from Papworth Hospital, Cambridge, and elsewhere have provided illustrations and other help and include: Dr David Hildick-Smith, Dr Peter Ludman, Mr Stephen Large, Mr John Dunning, Dr Michael Petch, Dr Leonard Shapiro, Dr David Stone, Dr Richard Coulden, Dr Edward Rowland, Dr Spencer Heald, Dr Mark Farrington, Dr Catherine Stephens, Mr John Wallwork, Mr Frank Wells and Professor John Jenkins. Medtronic Ltd and Guidant-CPI Ltd have also generously supplied illustrations. We would particularly like to thank the outstanding contribution made by Mr Stuart Newell. The assistance provided by the staff at the Medical Illustration department at Papworth hospital has been invaluable.

Contents

1 / Risk factors for coronary artery disease

Five principal risk factors have been identified for the development of atherosclerosis and coronary artery disease: male sex, increasing age, smoking, hyperlipidaemia and hypertension. The last three are reversible allowing the potential to reduce coronary risk.

Smoking

The risk of myocardial infarction in smokers is three times that of non-smokers. Stopping smoking leads to a reduction in risk and should be insisted on in all patients even in the absence of overt coronary artery disease (primary prevention).

Hyperlipidaemia

Raised plasma lipids are usually due to a combination of genetic (monogenic or polygenic) and environmental factors. Familial hypercholesterolaemia has been well characterized both clinically and at the molecular level and results in a raised plasma cholesterol, e.g. 8–15 mmol/l in heterozygotes (incidence approximately 1/500) associated with the early appearance of a corneal arcus, xanthelasma, tendon xanthomata and premature coronary artery disease. Homozygotes (incidence approximately 1 in 1 000 000) may have massively increased plasma cholesterol, e.g. 15–30 mmol/l with coronary artery disease usually first apparent in childhood.

Hypertension

Hypertension is an established strong independent risk for coronary artery disease. Disappointingly, in mild to moderate hypertension drug treatment results in a relatively minor reduction in the risk of MI (15%), compared to the reduction in the risk of stroke (40%).

Other risks

Patients with both insulin-dependent and non-insulin-dependent disease are at increased risk of developing macrovascular, and coronary artery, disease. Other markers of increased risk include raised fibrinogen levels, decreased serum TGFβ and the ACE DD genotype. Obesity, socio-economic factors and decreased physical activity have also been demonstrated to increase coronary risk but less so than the main factors identified above.

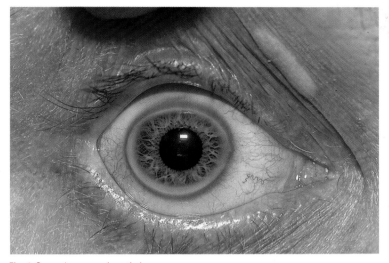

Fig. 1 Corneal arcus and xanthelasma.

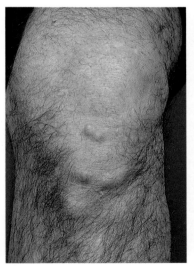

Fig. 2 Lipid deposition around the patella in type III hypercholesterolaemia.

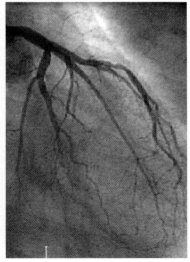

Fig. 3 Left coronary arteriogram from young patient with homozygous FH showing diffuse coronary disease.

2 / Angina pectoris

Angina pectoris is the usual symptomatic manifestation of myocardial ischaemia and results from obstructive coronary artery disease. Angina is most frequently described as a central substernal dull ache with radiation to the jaw and left arm. The most important feature to establish in the history is the relationship to exercise. The rapid resolution of symptoms on stopping exertion or with sublingual nitroglycerin is often the most important diagnostic clue. However, the clinical diagnosis is never simple with *atypical chest pain* being common and often difficult to distinguish from true angina.

Terminology

1. Chronic stable angina pectoris. Typical symptoms are predictably brought on by exercise or stress particularly in cold weather or after a heavy meal. Symptoms occur when myocardial oxygen demand outstrips supply, usually due to a fixed atheromatous narrowing impairing flow in one or more coronary arteries.

2. Unstable (crescendo) angina. Refers to a clinical syndrome (more akin to myocardial infarction than chronic stable angina) where angina occurs in a rapidly progressive pattern at rest or on minimal exertion. Referred to under an umbrella heading as an *acute coronary syndrome*.

3. Variant (Prinzmetal's) angina pectoris. Symptoms are essentially the same in character as in chronic stable angina but unpredictable in onset and unrelated to exertion. Thought to arise as a result of an increase in tone in a localized segment of the coronary arterial wall.

Pathology

Coronary narrowing due to atheroma is the most common cause of angina pectoris with symptoms usually appearing when coronary artery lesions become critical (usually >70% stenosis angiographically). Pathological studies however emphasise that even in the presence of such critical lesions patients may be asymptomatic with the initial manifestation being sudden death.

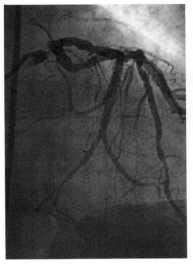

Fig. 4 Coronary arteriogram showing severe left main stem stenosis.

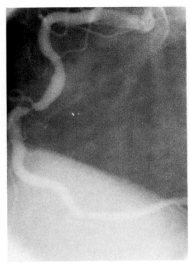

Fig. 5 Coronary stenosis in mid right coronary artery.

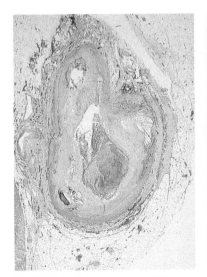

Fig. 6 Histological cross-section of an atheromatous plaque with luminal thrombus.

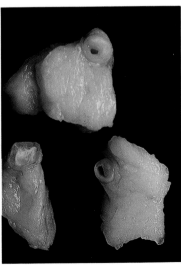

Fig. 7 Transverse sections through the three coronary arteries showing severe three vessel disease.

Angina pectoris (2)

Initial investigations

Electrocardiography. The initial assessment of the patient with symptoms suggestive of angina pectoris should include an ECG. In the majority of patients with uncomplicated angina the ECG is normal or there are minor non-specific repolarization (ST/T) changes. The best evidence for coronary artery disease in a patient with chest pain is the presence of Q waves corresponding to prior myocardial infarction (which may have been clinically silent).

Chest X-ray. This investigation is of little value in the patient with typical symptoms of angina; patients with coronary disease tend to have a normal chest X-ray unless there has been a previous myocardial infarction when the cardiac silhouette may occasionally be widened due to left ventricular dilatation. Another cause for angina pectoris may, however, be suggested by specific features, e.g. in aortic stenosis there may be valvular calcification seen best on the lateral projection.

Echocardiogram. Unnecessary in the majority of patients with uncomplicated angina but should be considered in some clinical situations, e.g. elderly patients with angina and a systolic murmur (could be aortic stenosis); with marked breathlessness or evidence of heart failure (could have left ventricular dysfunction which may be reversible).

Lipid profile. A random total cholesterol estimation is indicated in all patients with angina. A fasting sample should be obtained if the cholesterol is raised on initial estimation to allow more precise classification of the hyperlipidaemia and guide the selection of lipid-lowering therapy.

Further assessment

In most patients further investigations are required to establish the presence of underlying coronary artery disease and to stratify risk. These may be non-invasive usually involving some form of stress testing to establish the presence of reversible myocardial ischaemia. Invasive testing with coronary angiography can indicate both the presence and the extent of coronary artery disease.

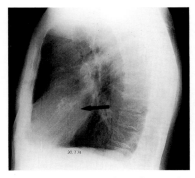

Fig. 8 Lateral chest X-ray in aortic stenosis showing valvar calcification.

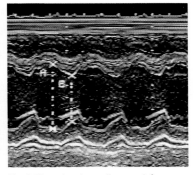

Fig. 9 M-mode echocardiogram, left ventricle showing impaired contraction.

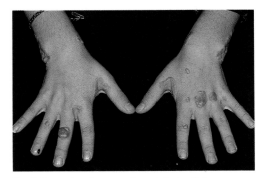

Fig. 10 Extensive planar xanthomata in familial hypercholesterolaemia.

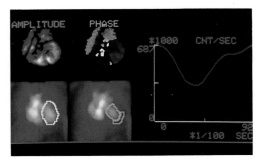

Fig. 11 Gated nuclear ventriculogram (MUGA) showing normal function (ejection fraction (EF) 53%) in a patient with angina.

Angina pectoris (3)

Exercise electrocardiography

Principal indications

1. To aid in diagnosis in patients presenting with atypical chest pain who have possible coronary artery disease. 2. To evaluate the extent of myocardial ischaemia and hence give some idea as to prognosis in patients with a clear diagnosis. Ideally most such patients under 70 years of age and selected older patients with a history of coronary artery disease should have an exercise electrocardiogram. 3. Risk stratification following myocardial infarction. 4. Provocation of arrhythmia in patients with palpitations provoked by exertion.

Contraindications

Most ambulant patients are capable of sufficient exercise to obtain a clinically useful result. In patients with unstable coronary disease, severe aortic stenosis or pulmonary hypertension the investigation is best avoided.

Method

Exercise level is gradually increased on a bicycle ergometer or motorised treadmill. Specific protocols allow comparison between centres and over time, e.g. the Bruce protocol.

Interpretation

In addition to the ECG, symptoms and the blood pressure response to exercise are observed. For exercise to be considered adequate the patient must have developed symptoms or ECG changes or reached the predetermined endpoint. The principal ECG change indicating a positive response is planar or down-sloping depression of the ST segment >0.1 mV (1 mm).

Myocardial perfusion imaging

Myocardial perfusion imaging employs exercise or pharmacological stress to provoke ischaemia. The isotope is injected at peak stress and its myocardial distribution relates to coronary flow. These tests can distinguish ischaemic (reversible defect) and infarcted tissue (irreversible defect) from normal tissue. Such *nuclear* investigations are indicated when there is diagnostic doubt following exercise ECG, in patients with an abnormal resting ECG in whom changes on exercise are not interpretable (bundle branch block, LVH etc.) and in patients, with, for example, peripheral vascular disease, who are unable to exercise.

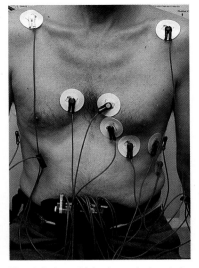

Fig. 12 Patient with leads attached ready for treadmill exercise test.

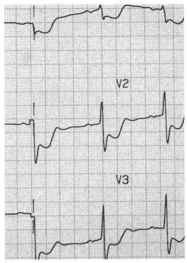

Fig. 13 Planar ST depression indicating myocardial ischaemia.

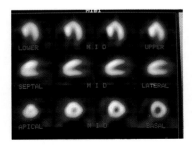

Fig. 14 Exercise perfusion study (rest image) showing normal perfusion.

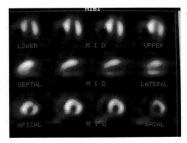

Fig. 15 Exercise perfusion study (exercise image) showing impaired segmental inferior perfusion.

Angina pectoris (4)

Coronary arteriography

With the development of more effective non-invasive methods of assessing the presence and extent of ischaemia cardiac catheterization is now principally indicated in patients with presumptive coronary artery disease to document the distribution of coronary narrowings and assess the need for revascularization. The development of percutaneous transluminal coronary angioplasty has widened the requirement for the technique and more than 600 000 angiograms are carried out annually in the United States.

Indications

Establishing the diagnosis.   In patients with atypical symptoms of angina pectoris and equivocal non-invasive investigations arteriography provides the only method of determining the diagnosis.

Determining prognosis.   In patients with evidence of readily provoked ischaemia, e.g. following myocardial infarction, arteriography allows optimal management. Prognosis is thought to be principally determined by the extent of coronary disease and left ventricular function.

Planning therapy.   In patients who have an inadequate response to drug therapy arteriography determines the most appropriate mode of revascularization.

Technique

The procedure is carried out under local anaesthetic. Arterial access is usually obtained via femoral or radial artery puncture or by cutdown onto the brachial artery. Pre-shaped catheters are used to selectively intubate the origins of the coronary arteries and enter the left ventricular cavity. Dye is injected through the lumen of the catheter and digital or cine images obtained. The procedure usually takes 5–10 min and is well tolerated by the majority of patients.

Complications

The incidence of major complications is approximately 0.24% with mortality about 0.06%. Most complications are produced at the site of vascular access (local complications).

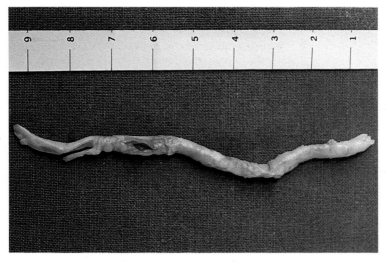

Fig. 16 Atheroma removed from coronary artery at endarterectomy.

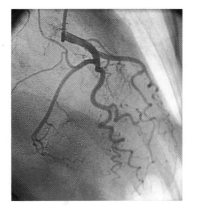

Fig. 17 Left coronary arteriogram.

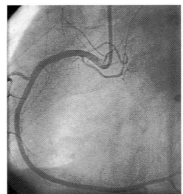

Fig. 18 Right coronary arteriogram.

Angina pectoris (5)

Management of angina
The main objectives in patients with angina are symptom relief, enhancement of prognosis and risk factor control. All patients should stop smoking, lose weight if obese and be encouraged to take regular exercise. Aspirin reduces the risk of myocardial infarction and should be given to all patients without contraindications. Medical therapy with sublingual nitrates, beta-blockers, calcium antagonists and long-acting oral nitrates is usually tried first. Hyperlipidaemia should be treated by diet, and drugs, e.g. statins, if necessary. Patients whose symptoms are inadequately relieved or who have prognostically severe disease, are candidates for *revascularization* with angioplasty or bypass surgery.

Percutaneous transluminal coronary angioplasty (PTCA)

Procedure

This procedure, like cardiac catheterization, is carried out under local anaesthetic. A fine guide wire is passed through the coronary catheter and down the coronary artery past the narrowing. A balloon catheter is passed over the guide wire and inflated, squashing the atheroma and stretching the artery, thus relieving the obstruction.

Results

Successful reduction of the coronary stenosis relieves angina. Studies comparing angioplasty with bypass surgery show, in general, a similar prognosis, but greater need for further revascularization procedures with angioplasty.

Problems

The mortality of coronary angioplasty is <1% with acute re-occlusion being the main concern. In 20–30% of patients *restenosis* of the dilated vessel occurs 1–6 months following coronary angioplasty.

Coronary stenting
Coronary stents are metallic coil or slotted tubular structures deployed by balloon inflation. Indications include acute occlusion or extensive dissection occurring during PTCA, restenosis, and vein graft disease. Stenting appears to reduce the risk of restenosis to 15–20%. The main risk is thrombotic occlusion, seen in around 4% of patients within 2 weeks.

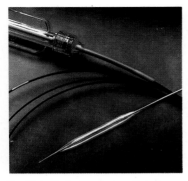

Fig. 19 Angioplasty catheter with balloon inflated.

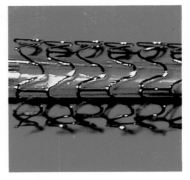

Fig. 20 Coronary stent.

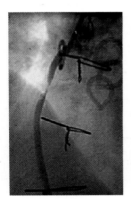

Fig. 21 Right coronary vein graft with severe stenosis.

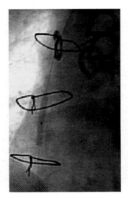

Fig. 22 Angioplasty balloon inflated at site of stenosis.

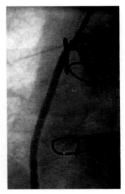

Fig. 23 Following balloon inflation the graft is widely patent.

Angina pectoris (6)

Coronary artery bypass surgery (CABG)

Indications

Relief of symptoms. CABG is an effective method of relieving angina with >90% success rate. In the United States patients with relatively mild symptoms are operated on; most patients in Europe have disabling symptoms or are intolerant of medical therapy. Coronary bypass surgery is the most common operation undertaken in the United States.

Improvement of prognosis. Patients with *left main stem* disease, many of those with *triple vessel disease* and some other subgroups have an improved prognosis following CABG. Contraindications to surgery are diminishing but risk increases with impaired left ventricular function and coexistent medical problems such as cerebrovascular disease.

Procedure

The left internal mammary artery (LIMA) is now the graft conduit of choice. It can however only be used for grafting one vessel usually the left anterior descending artery. Most patients require multiple bypasses and lengths of saphenous vein are used, anastomosed to the aortic root and to the distal segment of the diseased coronary arteries. Increasingly, other arterial conduits, e.g. radial arteries, are used as alternatives to vein grafts, because of their superior patency rates.

Risks

Perioperative mortality (1–2%) is not declining as patients with more preoperative risk factors become surgical candidates. Morbidity is low with the risk of significant post-bypass cerebral impairment being generally minor.

Follow-up

Coronary surgery remains palliative in the treatment of coronary disease. Patients require careful life-long follow-up with particular attention to secondary preventative measures. They should receive aspirin (if tolerated) and hyperlipidaemia should be vigorously controlled. Saphenous vein graft occlusion is inevitable and only lessened by these manoeuvres. LIMA grafts show a strikingly higher patency rate with prolonged relief of angina and improved prognosis.

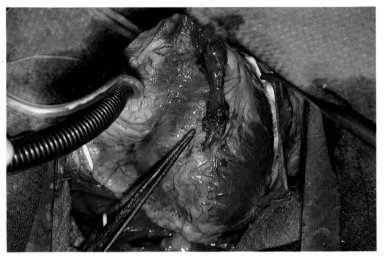

Fig. 24 Left internal mammary graft to LAD.

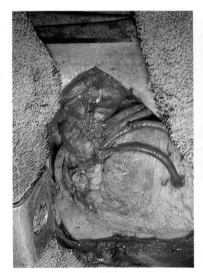

Fig. 25 Multiple saphenous vein grafts in situ.

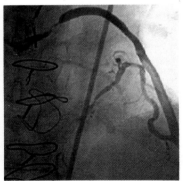

Fig. 26 Angiogram showing stenosed coronary artery saphenous vein graft.

3 / Variant angina pectoris

Definition

This rare condition is characterized by anginal pain occurring unpredictably at rest, often at night.

Pathophysiology

Increased tone in focal segments of a coronary artery (coronary vasoconstriction) leads to reduction in flow. The mechanism of vasospasm is not entirely clear but it may be associated with vasospasm elsewhere, e.g. Raynaud's phenomenon. It may however complicate coronary atherosclerosis producing a mixed picture with exercise-induced angina combined with some unpredictability in the precipitation of symptoms.

Investigations

Electrocardiography. ECG manifestations were first described by Prinzmetal (Prinzmetal's angina). During episodes of chest pain there is ST elevation (ST depression occurs with typical angina) returning to baseline as symptoms abate. Episodes of ischaemia may provoke ventricular arrhythmias often with a polymorphic pattern. ST segment change may occur in the absence of symptoms, as revealed by ambulatory ST segment monitoring.

Coronary arteriography may reveal normal coronary arteries with no evidence of obstructive disease. Coronary vasoconstriction (spasm) may be precipitated by the injection of ergonovine directly into the coronary artery lumen.

Management

The condition is unusual and optimal management is not established. The most common approach is to use coronary vasodilator agents especially calcium antagonists or nitrates often in high doses. Beta-blockers, in general, have adverse effects in the condition. In the presence of coexisting obstructive disease revascularization may be necessary.

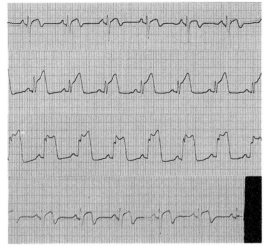

Fig. 27 ECG recorded in patient at rest showing periods of ST segment elevation associated with chest pain.

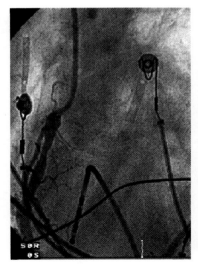

Fig. 28 Minor RCA stenosis.

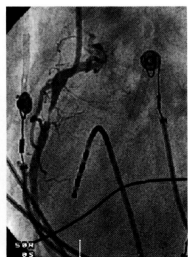

Fig. 29 Following injection of ergonovine the stenosis becomes critical.

16

4 / Unstable angina pectoris

Definition

Angina that is new or progresses rapidly is termed *unstable angina pectoris*.

Pathology

The underlying pathology is ulceration or rupture of an atheromatous plaque. Platelets adhere to the exposed collagen of the arterial wall narrowing the lumen. Cytokines are released increasing smooth muscle tone with vasoconstriction further reducing flow. The process has been most explicitly illustrated in vivo by angioscopy (using fibre-optic technology) but coronary arteriography usually also reveals eccentric lesions with ragged edges.

Investigations

Electrocardiography. An ECG during an episode of pain will often show ST depression with or without T wave inversion. Occasionally other patterns develop such as T wave peaking or bundle branch block.

Cardiac enzymes. A patient presenting with cardiac chest pain at rest without clear-cut ECG changes of infarction may have unstable angina, be developing a *non-Q wave* myocardial infarction or be in the very early stages of a *Q wave* myocardial infarction. These are distinguished by estimation of plasma levels of *cardiac* enzymes or subsequent ECG changes. Unstable angina is not associated with myocardial necrosis and there is no rise in *cardiac* enzymes. Other investigations are usually of little help although echocardiography may show wall motion abnormalities in the ischaemic zone.

Management

Unstable angina can usually be controlled with medical therapy. Standard regimens include oral aspirin, intravenous heparin and nitrates and oral beta-blockers and calcium antagonists. Acute intervention with angioplasty or coronary bypass may be required if symptoms prove refractory. Following resolution of the unstable phase exercise testing is indicated to assess subsequent prognosis. Coronary arteriography is indicated if non-invasive tests or continuing symptoms suggest severe coronary artery disease (as for chronic stable angina).

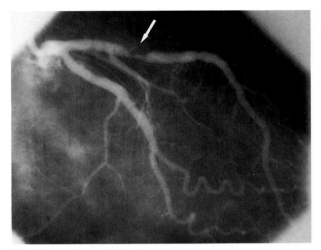

Fig. 30 Eccentric ragged LAD stenosis.

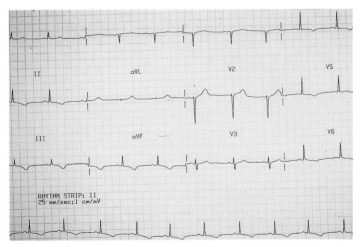

Fig. 31 ECG in unstable angina pectoris with widespread T wave inversion.

5 / Myocardial infarction

Incidence

Approximately 240 000 myocardial infarctions occur each year in the United Kingdom with the risk being approximately 1% per annum in middle-aged males. Primary Practitioners see on average 2–3 myocardial infarctions per year. Early recognition is required as 50% of all deaths occur within an hour of the onset of symptoms, but this can be reduced with appropriate management.

Pathology

Myocardial infarction is defined as myocardial necrosis following cessation of blood supply. The most common (>99%) cause of myocardial infarction is rupture or ulceration of an atheromatous plaque leading to localized thrombosis and coronary occlusion. Infarction is usually regional following the occlusion of a single coronary artery. Two patterns are described with either the full thickness of the myocardium involved or necrosis localized to the subendocardium. Histological changes are not apparent for 12 h following coronary occlusion and this has given impetus to the optimization of treatment designed to achieve early reopening of acutely occluded coronary arteries.

Diagnosis

The diagnosis of myocardial infarction revolves on three criteria: history, ECG and cardiac enzymes.

History. A typical history is available from most patients with crushing retrosternal chest pain associated with shortness of breath, sweating, nausea and vomiting. The pain may radiate to the jaw and arms and typically builds up over several minutes. Symptoms in older patients may be atypical and not immediately referable to the heart; for example myocardial infarction may present as an acute confusional state. Under such conditions retrospective recognition is often all that is available and myocardial infarction is described as *silent* (20–30% of total). It is important to review very carefully the differential diagnosis (e.g. dissecting aneurysm, gastrointestinal catastrophe etc.) especially if thrombolytics are considered.

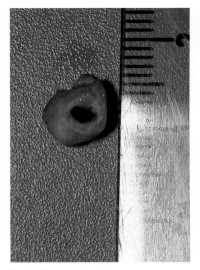

Fig. 32 Cross-section of postmortem specimen of the LAD showing the cause of MI: intraluminal thrombus.

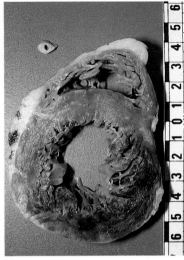

Fig. 33 Macroscopic image showing extensive transmural MI with haemorrhage and necrosis.

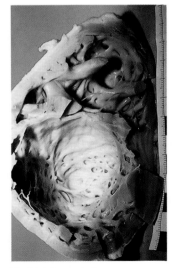

Fig. 34 Left ventricular aneurysm following full thickness myocardial infarction.

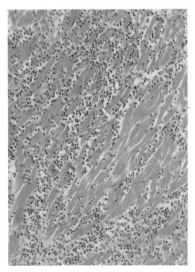

Fig. 35 Neutrophilic infiltrate in the myocardium in acute MI.

Myocardial infarction (2)

Diagnosis
(contd.)

Electrocardiography.   It is essential to record a 12-lead ECG in patients in whom the diagnosis is considered. ST elevation is the first change supporting the diagnosis of myocardial infarction (Q waves and T wave inversion develop later) and T wave changes in isolation may be suggestive but are not diagnostic. Evolving myocardial infarction with pain is usually associated with ECG changes— chest pain and a normal ECG should suggest either alternative possible diagnoses (e.g. dissecting aortic aneurysm, Fig. 38) or a request for serial ECGs. In patients with chest pain and regional ST elevation >1 mm in the limb leads or >2 mm in the precordial leads the diagnosis of myocardial infarction is virtually certain and specific therapy should be initiated without delay.

Enzymes.   Serial blood samples for enzyme estimation are usually taken and help to establish the diagnosis of myocardial infarction. CK-MB fraction, myoglobin and troponin are more recently introduced enzyme markers of myocardial damage and are usually elevated prior to older established markers (e.g. CK, AST and LDH).

Plasma lipids.   Myocardial infarction is often the first manifestation of coronary artery disease and blood obtained from the patient should be sent for lipid analysis. The results should, however, be interpreted with caution as the stress of myocardial infarction will influence measured values.

Further
investigations

Echocardiography.   In patients with uncomplicated myocardial infarction echocardiography is not necessary. In those patients with cardiogenic shock, pulmonary oedema, new murmurs etc. echocardiography may be essential.

Right heart catheterization.   Invasive monitoring of right heart pressures and pulmonary capillary wedge pressure (an index of the left heart filling pressures) by insertion of a Swan–Ganz catheter is not required in uncomplicated myocardial infarction. However, in patients with complications, e.g. shock, such information may occasionally be considered useful.

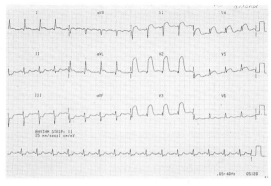

Fig. 36 ECG showing changes of hyperacute anterior MI.

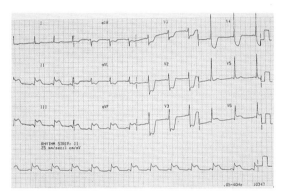

Fig. 37 Early change inferior and posterior MI.

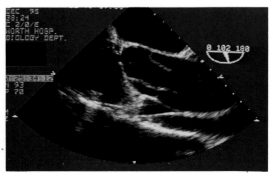

Fig. 38 Transoesophageal echo of acute aortic dissection.

Myocardial infarction (3)

General management

Management of acute myocardial infarction has seen dramatic changes in recent years and now more than ever speed in diagnosis and management are essential. Health education should encourage the public to summon help immediately for patients with suspected myocardial infarction, as at present relatives take an average of 90 min to call for help. If myocardial infarction is suspected patients should be admitted to a coronary care unit.

Initial management. A defibrillator should be available as the incidence of serious ventricular arrhythmias is highest during the early phases with 25% of deaths occurring before the patient reaches hospital. Intravenous analgesia along with an antiemetic should be administered and oxygen given if available. Aspirin should be given unless contraindicated.

Thrombolysis

Thrombolytic drugs can reopen an occluded coronary artery by *lysing* occlusive thrombus with reperfusion of the myocardium distal to the occlusion reducing infarct size. Several large-scale clinical studies have now conclusively shown that the early administration of an intravenous thrombolytic agent improves prognosis.

Indications

Provided there are no contraindications thrombolytics should be given to all patients with cardiac chest pain and ST elevation or new bundle branch block seen within 12 h of the onset of symptoms. In patients in whom the diagnosis is in doubt, e.g. no ECG changes or non-specific findings (ST depression, T wave changes) thrombolytic therapy should be withheld and the patient observed with serial ECGs.

Choice of agent

Tissue plasminogen activator (tPA) may be given in preference to streptokinase for large (usually anterior) infarcts. Streptokinase should not be given if it has been administered in the preceding year as antistreptokinase antibodies associated with allergic responses and decreased efficacy may be present. Intravenous heparin and beta-blockers may also be administered.

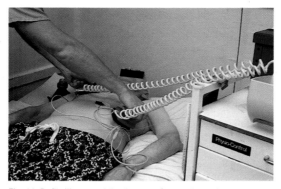

Fig. 39 Defibrillator paddles in place for cardioversion.

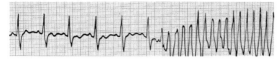

Fig. 40 Rhythm strip showing sinus rhythm degenerating to ventricular tachycardia.

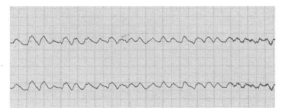

Fig. 41 Ventricular fibrillation.

Myocardial infarction (4)

Contraindications

Thrombolysis
In general it is unsafe to give thrombolytic therapy to patients with a recent history of haemorrhagic stroke, peptic ulceration or recent gastrointestinal surgery, a bleeding diathesis, severe hypertension or during pregnancy. Proliferative diabetic retinopathy is a relative contraindication. Careful assessment of the history and ECG should identify those patients with aortic dissection or other causes of chest pain.

Complications

The major complication is bleeding. Even superficial bruising following vascular puncture may be severe but more worrying is gastrointestinal blood loss or intracranial haemorrhage. Other problems include those due to hypersensitivity following streptokinase, e.g. anaphylaxis, rashes, proteinuria, and a serum sickness like illness. As currently used the benefits of thrombolytic therapy far outweigh these potential risks.

Mechanical revascularization
Routine angioplasty following thrombolysis is not beneficial, but there is a role for *rescue* PTCA in patients with persistent coronary occlusion or cardiogenic shock. *Primary* PTCA (angioplasty without antecedent thrombolysis) has been shown to improve coronary artery patency, LV function and mortality, but requires on-site cardiac catheterization facilities and has significant staffing implications.

Prognosis following myocardial infarction
There are three major determinants of survival following myocardial infarction namely residual left ventricular function, the extent of the underlying coronary disease and the degree of electrical instability. Full assessment of the patient includes consideration of each of these features prior to discharge (risk stratification). The measures taken depend on the institution but should include an echocardiogram and an exercise test.

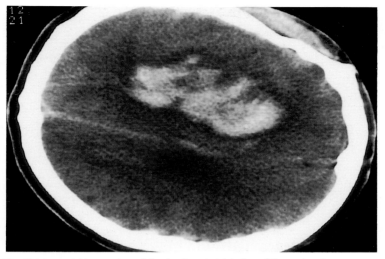

Fig. 42 Intracranial haemorrhage following the administration of tissue plasminogen activator (t-PA).

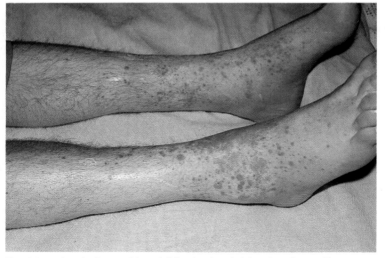

Fig. 43 Leucocytoclastic vasculitic rash following the administration of streptokinase.

Myocardial infarction (5)

Complications

Arrhythmias

Many arrhythmias can complicate acute myocardial infarction. Ventricular extrasystoles are very common (>90%) and, in general, do not require treatment. Reperfusion following thrombolysis may lead to transient sinus bradycardia or slow idioventricular rhythms which can be treated conservatively. Tachyarrhythmias, often ventricular in origin usually require immediate intervention. Complete heart block associated with inferior myocardial infarction is usually transient. Complete heart block with anterior myocardial infarction is associated with large infarcts and will probably require permanent pacing if the patient survives.

Mechanical complications

The presentation of mechanical complications of acute myocardial infarction is usually with shock (circulatory collapse and pulmonary oedema).

Cardiogenic shock. Associated with extensive myocardial infarction (>40% of LV mass). The incidence remains around 5% and mortality >75%.

Ventricular septal defect/Acute mitral regurgitation. Suggested by a new systolic murmur in a shocked patient. Diagnosis is made with echocardiography and Doppler. Surgical repair offers the best chance of survival; however mortality remains around 50%.

Ventricular free wall rupture. Causes 10% of in-hospital deaths following myocardial infarction reduced by early administration of intravenous beta-blockers. Mortality approaches 100%. Immediate surgical repair offers the only chance of survival.

Pericarditis. Acute pericarditis with chest pain and pericardial rub may occur with transmural infarction. Dressler syndrome (fever, pericarditis, raised ESR) may appear 2–10 weeks following myocardial infarction.

Left ventricular aneurysm. Develops in up to 10% of patients and aneurysmectomy may be required in patients with intractable heart failure.

Left ventricular thrombus. Detected by echo (20–40% of anterior infarcts). Embolism may cause stroke or peripheral arterial occlusion.

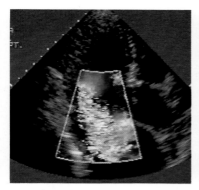

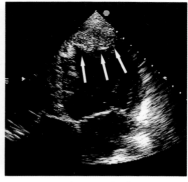

Fig. 44 Colour flow Doppler showing acute MR with jet demonstrated from the LV to the left atrium.

Fig. 45 Apical left ventricular thrombus.

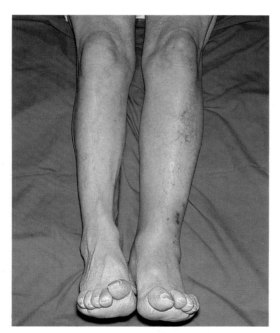

Fig. 46 Prolonged immobility following MI may lead to venous thrombosis with the risk of pulmonary embolism.

6 / Acute heart failure

Definition

Acute heart failure is a sudden decline in left ventricular function usually resulting in both high filling pressures and a low cardiac output. In most patients a vicious circle of events is established where a decline in cardiac function leads to pulmonary oedema with hypoxia and hypotension, both of which cause a fall in myocardial perfusion and further deterioration in cardiac pumping ability.

Aetiology

Acute heart failure usually arises as a result of acute myocardial infarction and such patients will have extensive left ventricular damage and a poor prognosis, unless an acute mechanical complication has occurred which is surgically correctable (Figs 47–50). In patients with chronic left ventricular disease, an arrhythmia or other circulatory stress (e.g. infection, anaemia, minor pulmonary embolus, thyrotoxicosis) may precipitate acute heart failure. Myocarditis may present with severe heart failure and a potentially fatal course. The diagnosis of pericardial effusion with tamponade should always be considered in patients presenting with this clinical picture since it is readily treatable by pericardial drainage.

Presentation

An acute onset of shortness of breath leads to patient discomfort and restlessness. Chest pain and palpitation may accompany dyspnoea and provide a useful clue to the underlying mechanism. The clinical appearance is characteristic with the patient sitting upright and using the accessory muscles of respiration. The skin is pale, cool and moist. Consciousness may be impaired.

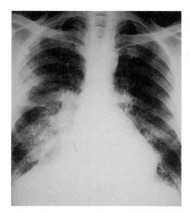

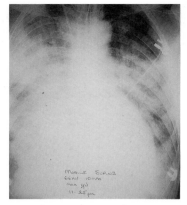

Fig. 47 Mitral valve rupture following MI showing pulmonary oedema.

Fig. 48 Same patient as in Fig. 45 showing extent of deterioration 4 h later.

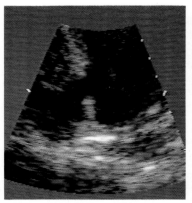

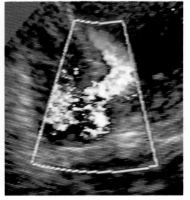

Fig. 49 Ventricular septal defect on two-dimensional echo.

Fig. 50 Colour flow across defect.

Acute heart failure (2)

There is usually a tachycardia, and hypotension with cool extremities due to intense vasoconstriction. Third and fourth heart sounds are common and the jugular venous pressure may be raised. The presence of murmurs may suggest a specific cause but basal crackles lack both sensitivity and specificity in the diagnosis of pulmonary oedema. Oliguria is usual.

Investigations

Chest X-ray. Usually shows changes of pulmonary oedema with septal lines (Kerley B lines). The heart may be enlarged and evidence of a valve lesion may be present. A large globular heart shadow should suggest the possibility of a pericardial effusion.

Electrocardiogram. Useful in elucidating arrhythmias and establishing a diagnosis of myocardial infarction.

Echocardiogram. An early echocardiogram may help to diagnose the cause of heart failure and exclude pericardial effusion. An assessment of left ventricular function can be made.

Haemodynamic monitoring. Patients not responding rapidly to treatment may benefit from invasive monitoring. An arterial line to monitor systemic arterial pressure is useful but a Swan–Ganz balloon flotation catheter to measure ventricular filling pressures should only be used if there is a clear indication of potential benefit.

Management

General. Oxygen should be administered and assisted ventilation may be required. Intravenous diamorphine relieves distress and causes venodilation (reducing preload). Specific management is determined by the initial assessment and may include intravenous frusemide and nitrates to reduce preload, correction of any arrhythmia and positive inotropes for hypotension. Intra-aortic balloon counter-pulsation may be required. In patients with surgically correctable lesions early referral to a regional cardiothoracic centre is essential.

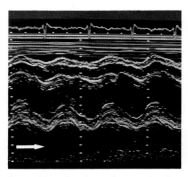

Fig. 51 M-mode echocardiogram showing large pericardial effusion (echo-free space around heart).

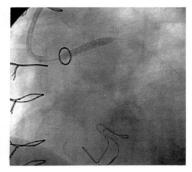

Fig. 52 Acute revascularization using PTCA in patient with cardiogenic shock due to acute vein graft occlusion.

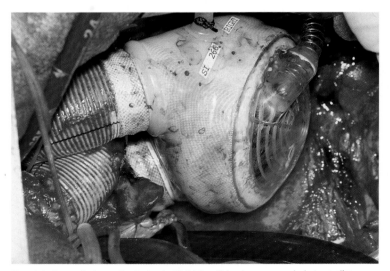

Fig. 53 Left ventricular assist device (artificial heart) in place as a prelude to cardiac transplantation.

7 / Chronic heart failure

Definition

The definition of chronic heart failure remains contentious but has been described as *left ventricular dysfunction with symptoms*. Heart failure is not a diagnosis but a complex of symptoms with evidence of ventricular disease and a specific aetiology should be established. The prevalence in Europe is around 0.45% overall rising to 3% in elderly patients. 10% of people over the age of 75 are thought to have heart failure.

Aetiology

Coronary artery disease. Responsible for 50–75% of cases. Usually due to left ventricular damage from prior myocardial infarction. Some patients with severe coronary artery disease and no evidence of previous myocardial infarction may have ventricular dysfunction (hibernating myocardium) that is improved by revascularization.

Dilated cardiomyopathy accounts for the majority of the remainder (20–30% of cases).

Hypertension was previously quoted as the most common cause of heart failure but is now uncommon (<5%). Others causes, e.g. myocarditis, valvular heart disease, restrictive cardiomyopathy and hypertrophic cardiomyopathy, are also uncommon (<5% in total).

Pathophysiology

Systolic heart failure. The primary defect in the majority of patients is impaired cardiac contractility. Compensatory mechanisms may be initially helpful but ultimately contribute to the progression of heart failure and worsening symptoms. Therapy in heart failure is currently directed to countering these compensatory effects, e.g. by using angiotensin-converting-enzyme (ACE) inhibitors.

Diastolic heart failure. The primary defect in other patients with heart failure, e.g. with LVH, is impaired ventricular relaxation. The relative components of diastolic and systolic dysfunction in any particular patient are important to establish, e.g. with echo/Doppler to guide therapy.

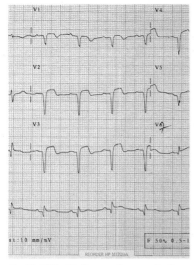

Fig. 54 ECG with Q waves in many leads indicating extensive myocardial damage.

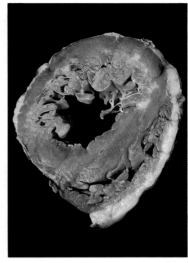

Fig. 55 Extensive old anterior myocardial infarction.

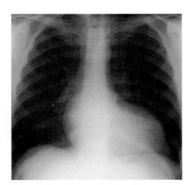

Fig. 56 Chest X-ray showing the appearances of a left ventricular aneurysm.

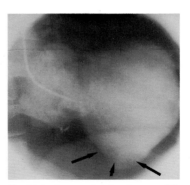

Fig. 57 Angiogram showing the same LV aneurysm as a large akinetic segment.

Chronic heart failure (2)

Assessment

The assessment of a patient with heart failure should determine the likely aetiology, its clinical severity, the likely rate of progression, identify any surgically remediable disease, and plan therapy.

Symptoms

Principal symptoms relate to fluid retention with dyspnoea, orthopnoea and ankle swelling. Symptoms of reduced cardiac output with lethargy, fatigue and cognitive impairment may also be prominent if sought.

Signs

A group of signs are conventionally accepted as being indicative of the presence of ventricular failure (tachycardia, displacement of the apex beat, added third and fourth heart sounds) or represent compensatory fluid retention (raised venous pressure, peripheral oedema, basal crackles, palpable liver edge). None of these signs give any clue as to the underlying cause. Heart murmurs may identify valvular disease amenable to surgery, e.g. aortic stenosis or mitral regurgitation.

Investigations

Chest X-ray. Any patient with breathlessness or a raised venous pressure should have a chest X-ray. The important observations in heart failure are the heart size and the presence or absence of pulmonary oedema. The presence of underlying valvular heart disease or congenital heart disease may also be highlighted.

Electrocardiogram. In patients with heart failure an ECG often provides important clues to the likely aetiology (previous myocardial infarction) and will identify rhythm disturbances.

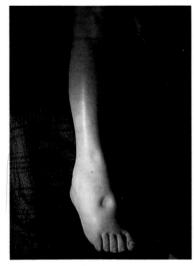

Fig. 58 Pitting oedema.

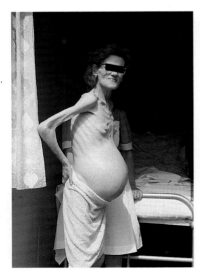

Fig. 59 Ascites associated with severe heart failure and tricuspid regurgitation.

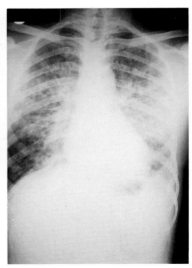

Fig. 60 Pulmonary oedema with normal heart size.

Chronic heart failure (3)

Investigations (cont.)

Echocardiography. All patients with heart failure should have a baseline echocardiogram to assess left ventricular function and exclude a potentially surgically correctable cause.

Nuclear ventriculography remains the best way of obtaining a non-invasive quantitative measure of left ventricular function. The result is often expressed as the ejection fraction (%) and the test also allows an estimation of localized heart function. Wall motion abnormalities may be seen in coronary artery disease. The presence of a left ventricular aneurysm may be detected and suggest possible benefit from surgery. *Magnetic resonance imaging* (MRI) provides detailed information on global and localized LV function.

Myocardial perfusion imaging. Some patients with coronary disease may benefit from revascularization, if metabolic studies, e.g. positron emission tomography (PET), demonstrate viable (*hibernating*) myocardium.

Prognosis

The two main predictors of outcome are left ventricular function and the presence of arrhythmia. Much of the prognostic data however relates to symptomatic status. Patients with symptoms on mild exertion or at rest (New York Heart Association (NYHA) class 3–4) have an annual mortality of approximately 30–40%. This figure is comparable to many cancers. The majority of patients however die suddenly and have been generally assumed to have an arrhythmia as the agonal event. The presence of an arrhythmia on ambulatory electrocardiograms correlates with increased risk but suppression of these arrhythmias does not appear to improve prognosis particularly if cardiac failure is the result of myocardial infarction.

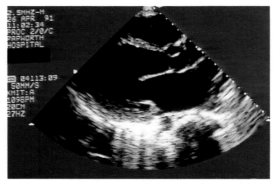

Fig. 61 Two-dimensional echocardiogram showing poor left ventricular function (diastolic frame).

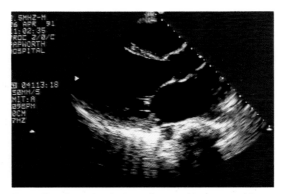

Fig. 62 Two-dimensional echocardiogram showing poor left ventricular function (systolic frame).

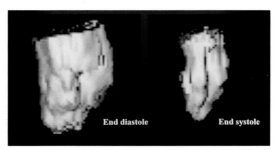

End diastole   End systole

Fig. 63 MRI three-dimensional reconstruction to assess LV function.

Chronic heart failure (4)

Medical therapy

The principal aims of treatment are to control symptoms and hence enhance quality of life, and to improve survival. General advice should include moderate exercise that helps to prevent deconditioning and may improve outlook, cessation of smoking, and reduction of alcohol and salt intake. Drugs include:

1. *Diuretics* are the first step in most patients and improve symptoms but have no described beneficial effect on prognosis. With careful use side-effects are relatively infrequent.
2. *Digoxin* is indicated in patients in atrial fibrillation. The benefits in sinus rhythm remain controversial and digoxin is not usually considered first-line therapy.
3. *ACE inhibitors* are the mainstay of treatment and have the advantage that they improve both symptoms and prognosis in most patients. However they should be used with caution in patients with coexistent peripheral vascular disease, as in those with renal artery disease precipitation of acute renal failure may occur.
4. *Beta-blockers* may reverse some of the adverse effects of chronic sympathetic stimulation.

Cardiac transplantation

In some patients with end-stage heart failure transplantation will provide the most effective means of usefully improving symptoms and prognosis. The resource however is limited by the size of the donor pool. Immunosuppressive treatment usually with cyclosporine A, azathioprine and prednisolone is required. Currently, at Papworth Hospital, the one year survival following cardiac transplantation is 89%. Deaths in the first year are usually due to acute rejection and infection but after the first year survival is usually maintained for 8–10 years. Left ventricular assist devices, mechanical pumps that extract blood directly from the left ventricle and deliver it to the proximal aorta can be implanted surgically as a bridge to transplantation, and are also being assessed for more chronic use. Xeno-transplantation may increase the supply of donor hearts in the future.

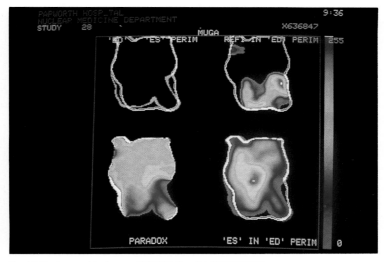

Fig. 64 Nuclear ventriculogram (MUGA) showing LV aneurysm.

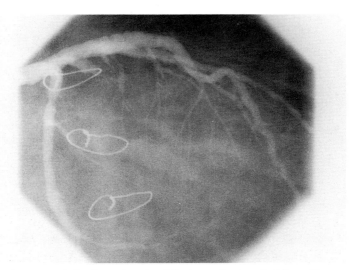

Fig. 65 Coronary occlusive disease in patient following cardiac transplantation, with tapered vessels and absent side branches.

Dilated (congestive) cardiomyopathy is defined as left ventricular dilatation with systolic dysfunction in the absence of coronary artery disease, valvular heart disease and hypertension.

Aetiology

In most patients a precise cause for dilated cardiomyopathy cannot be established. It is thought that many cases follow an episode (often subclinical) of viral myocarditis, e.g. Coxsackie infection. Excessive alcohol consumption may lead to dilated cardiomyopathy with other specific causes including nutritional deficiencies (thiamine, selenium), toxins (doxorubicidin, cobalt), specific viral infections (HIV), infiltrations (sarcoidosis, haemochromatosis) and thyroid disease. Peripartum cardiomyopathy is a rare cause, which usually occurs in late pregnancy or the puerperium.

Investigations

Electrocardiogram. Non-specific repolarization changes bundle branch block and atrial and ventricular arrhythmias are common.

Chest X-ray. Cardiomegaly is usually present. Pulmonary oedema is also seen.

Echocardiography. Characteristic features are of a poorly functioning dilated left ventricle in the absence of regional wall motion abnormalities.

Cardiac catheterization will exclude coronary artery disease and *endomyocardial biopsy* is a relatively easy method of obtaining a sample of ventricular myocardium for histology.

Therapy

As for heart failure. Anticoagulation protects against systemic embolism. In selected patients beneficial effects with beta-blockers have been reported but immunosuppressive therapy appears to be of no overall benefit.

Prognosis

Difficult to predict in individual patients, with a 50% mortality in the first 2 years following diagnosis but with 25% of patients surviving >10 years.

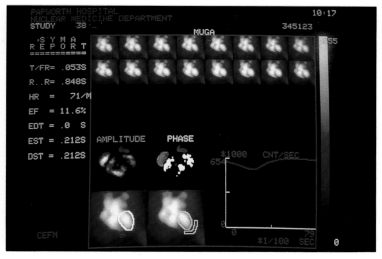

MUGA

S Y M A
R E P O R T
==========

T/FR= .053S

R..R= .848S

HR =   71/M

EF = 11.6%

EDT = .0 S

EST = .212S   AMPLITUDE   PHASE

DST = .212S

Fig. 66 Gated nuclear ventriculogram showing impaired left ventricular function (EF 11.6%) in dilated cardiomyopathy.

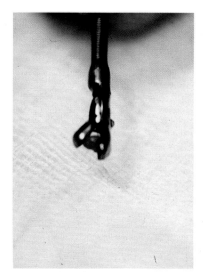

Fig. 67 Endomyocardial biopsy forceps with specimen of right ventricular myocardium.

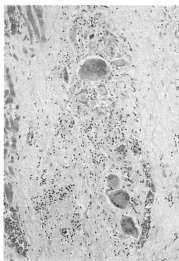

Fig. 68 Sarcoid granulomas from biopsy specimen in patient with dilated cardiomyopathy.

Myocarditis

Acute inflammatory disease of the myocardium is usually due to infection with viruses (Coxsackie, echo) but occasionally other causes such as drug hypersensitivity or allergy (toxic myocarditis) are present. Clinical manifestations are variable with heart failure, chest pain and arrhythmias. Occasionally there is an acute presentation with rapidly progressive heart failure or shock. Treatment is largely symptomatic with diuretics and ACE-inhibitors and if necessary inotropic and mechanical support. Spontaneous resolution may occur leading to dramatic recovery. Cardiac transplantation improves the outlook in selected cases, although the use of this rare resource in sick ventilated patients receiving inotropic support is controversial. There is no reduction in mortality from immunosuppressive treatment.

Restrictive cardiomyopathy

Rare condition characterized by a thickened and stiff left ventricle with impaired diastolic filling. Systolic function is usually well preserved. No specific cause is established in the majority of patients but the condition may be due to endomyocardial fibrosis, infiltration with amyloid, sarcoid, or by haemochromatosis. Patients present with heart failure symptoms and a chest X-ray showing normal heart size but pulmonary oedema with appearances that may be confused with primary lung disease such as fibrosing alveolitis. The diagnosis is often first suggested by echocardiography but the differentiation from constrictive pericarditis which has a similar clinical presentation is difficult and important. Distinguishing the two may require endomyocardial biopsy and CT scanning or magnetic resonance imaging (MRI). Medical therapy is difficult. Over-diuresis must be avoided, and cardiac transplantation may be needed.

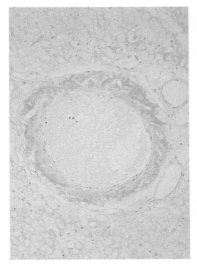

Fig. 69 Endomyocardial biopsy specimen showing amyloid (congo red).

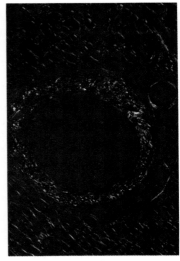

Fig. 70 Endocardial biopsy specimen showing amyloid (congo repolarized).

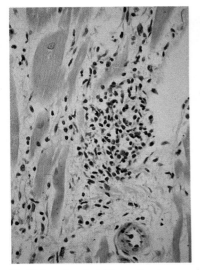

Fig. 71 Lymphocytic infiltrate of acute myocarditis.

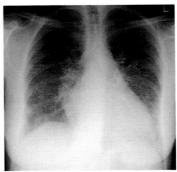

Fig. 72 Chest X-ray from patient with restrictive cardiomyopathy.

Definition

Heart muscle disease with unexplained ventricular hypertrophy. Symptoms are due to obstruction of left ventricular outflow and impaired ventricular relaxation. 60% of cases are familial and approximately 40% occur sporadically. Transmitted as autosomal dominant with many mutations of the β-myosin heavy chain, troponin T and α tropomyosin genes described. Screening and risk stratification on the basis of mutation type or echo cardiography has been advocated.

Clinical picture

Chest pain, dyspnoea, syncope and sudden death may be prominent but patients are often asymptomatic. Examination findings include a jerky carotid upstroke, palpable atrial thrust, 4th heart sound and a harsh ejection systolic murmur.

Investigations

Electrocardiography. Often very abnormal with left ventricular hypertrophy, bundle branch block, large septal *q* waves and repolarization changes.

Chest X-ray. Often normal. Cardiomegaly and occasionally, pulmonary oedema may be seen.

Echocardiogram. Diagnostic. Asymmetric hypertrophy of the ventricular septum is often seen but other distinct patterns of hypertrophy, e.g. concentric, are described.

Ambulatory ECG. Indicated in all patients to establish the presence of asymptomatic ventricular arrhythmias. Non-sustained ventricular tachycardia is a predictor of risk of sudden death, which occurs in 2–4% of adult patients per year.

Therapy

Symptoms may improve with calcium antagonists, beta-blockers or disopyramide. Diuretics and vasodilators may have adverse symptomatic effects and digoxin is, in general, contraindicated. Amiodarone for patients with non-sustained ventricular tachycardia may improve prognosis. Dual-chamber pacing can improve symptoms in some patients. Surgery (myomectomy and/or mitral valve replacement) is occasionally required.

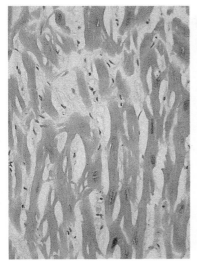

Fig. 73 Histology showing the myocyte disarray in hypertrophic cardiomyopathy.

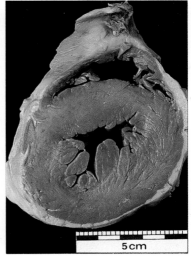

Fig. 74 Concentric hypertrophic cardiomyopathy.

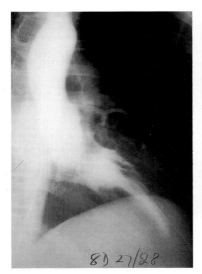

Fig. 75 Left ventricular angiogram showing characteristic appearances of hypertrophic cardiomyopathy with papillary muscle thickening.

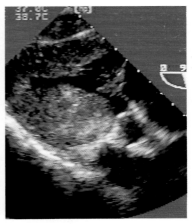

Fig. 76 Echocardiogram showing severe hypertrophy.

Aetiology

An increase in left ventricular mass in the absence of valvular disease may occur in patients with elevated blood pressure, increasing age, obesity, and in men, physical activity. Primary genetic disease, e.g. hypertrophic cardiomyopathy, Fabry's disease, should always be considered but the cause may not be identified even after extensive investigation. The incidence of left ventricular hypertrophy (LVH) in the general population based on ECG recordings is 2.1%, but echocardiographic evidence of LVH has been found in up to 16%.

LVH in hypertension

LVH in hypertension is both an adaptive response to increased work and an adverse prognostic indicator. Hypertrophy is usually concentric with an increase in wall thickness and no increase in chamber size. ECG evidence of LVH is found in 15% of unselected patients with mild hypertension, 50% of patients with mild to moderate hypertension and 90% of patients admitted to hospital with hypertension. LVH is 10 times more prevalent in patients with blood pressure >160/95 than in the normotensive population.

Athlete's heart

The adaptive LVH that occurs with endurance training is difficult to distinguish morphologically from pathological LVH, although hypertrophy due to training resolves on cessation of athletic activity. LV wall thickness in excess of 1.3 cm has been found in rowers and cyclists, and ECG criteria for LVH are present in 85% of endurance athletes. Sudden death in the setting of *physiological* LVH is rare and in those instances where young athletes die suddenly there is usually evidence of underlying heart disease such as hypertrophic cardiomyopathy or coronary disease. The value of screening for such abnormalities in athletes is not clear.

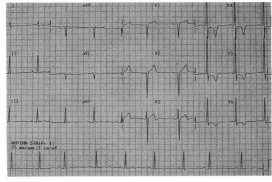

Fig. 77 ECG in LVH showing tall R waves and T wave inversion.

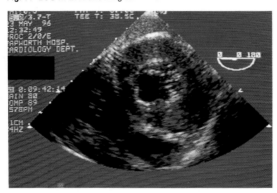

Fig. 78 Echocardiogram in LVH. Heart is seen in transverse plane with small ventricular cavity.

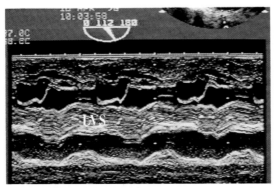

Fig. 79 M-mode echocardiogram showing severe septal hypertrophy in an athlete with hypertropic cardiomyopathy.

Left ventricular hypertrophy (2)

Clinical picture

Most patients are asymptomatic. Exertional dyspnoea, the most common symptom, is a consequence of impaired relaxation and filling of a stiff ventricle. Angina may occur even in patients without coronary disease, because of increased LV muscle mass, and decreased coronary flow reserve. Palpitations may occur because of ventricular ectopy. Examination may reveal a sustained cardiac impulse, and audible 4th heart sound.

Consequences

The presence of LVH increases the risk of fatal events in both male and female patients with hypertension and in men aged 35–64 increases risk more than sevenfold. Initially systolic function is well maintained, but in time hypertrophy leads to impairment of relaxation and heart failure which in hypertension is the result of increased workload, direct myocyte necrosis and decreases in coronary vascular reserve. The incidence of heart failure arising as a consequence of hypertension has decreased dramatically probably as a function of improved detection and treatment of hypertension. When hypertension is due to phaechromocytoma then sudden surges of blood pressure may lead to acute heart failure.

Detection

Electrocardiography. Standard method of detection. Electrocardiography has a sensitivity of only 50%, but a specificity of 90%. Standard criteria sum voltages from R wave in V_1 or V_2 and S wave in V_5 or V_6 which should not exceed 35 mm. Repolarization changes commonly accompany these changes.

Echocardiography. Echocardiography has the highest sensitivity and specificity. Increased wall thickness or muscle mass on echo is now taken as the standard index of LVH for epidemiological or clinical studies.

Treatment

Control of hypertension by most antihypertensive drugs, reduces LVH, but calcium antagonists and ACE inhibitors appear to have greatest effect. There is some evidence that regression of LVH reduces the frequency of ventricular arrhythmias, but it is not clear whether this results in a reduction of the risk of sudden death.

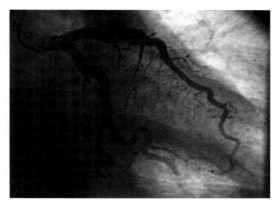

Fig. 80 Normal left coronary artery in a patient with LVH and angina.

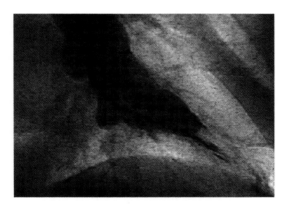

Fig. 81 Supra-normal systolic function on LV angiography.

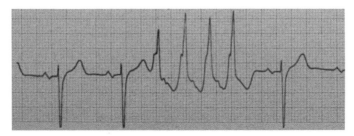

Fig. 82 Ventricular ectopy in LVH.

Aetiology

Congenital. 1–2% population have a bicuspid aortic valve. The valve may degenerate with calcification in adult life leading to aortic stenosis and/or regurgitation. Congenital aortic stenosis may be valvular, subvalvular, or supravalvular. Aortic stenosis may occur as an isolated abnormality or be associated with a typical *elfin* facies, mental retardation and hypercalcaemia (William syndrome). Both these forms are due to mutations in the gene encoding elastin.

Degenerative. *Calcific* aortic stenosis is the most common symptomatic valve lesion seen in adults. Approximately 50% arise secondary to a bicuspid aortic valve.

Rheumatic. Isolated rheumatic aortic valve disease is now relatively rare and is usually *mixed* (95%) with stenotic and regurgitant components. Coexistent mitral valve disease is usual.

Symptoms

The three classic symptoms of aortic stenosis are angina, dyspnoea and syncope. The symptoms are non-specific often leading to delayed diagnosis. Angina may occur with normal coronary arteries as a result of increased ventricular mass but in older patients coronary artery disease is frequently present.

Signs

The most important signs are a slow rising carotid arterial pulse; a sustained apical impulse and a systolic murmur in the aortic area radiating to the neck, but often loudest at the apex (*Gallavardin phenomenon*). Clinical signs can give an approximate indication of the severity of the disease. Clinical assessment must therefore be confirmed using other tests particularly echo-Doppler. Hypertension in older patients with aortic stenosis is not uncommon and the pulse pressure may be wide in view of the rigid peripheral circulation. Systolic pressures of greater than 200 mm Hg are however unusual in patients with critical aortic stenosis.

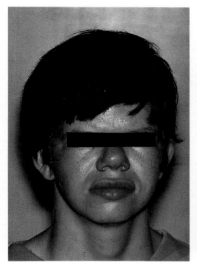

Fig. 83 Facies of supravalvar aortic stenosis.

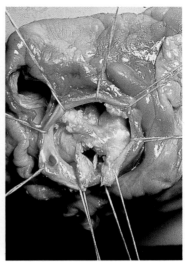

Fig. 84 Pathology of calcific aortic stenosis.

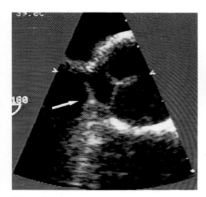

Fig. 85 Transoesophageal echo showing subvalvar aortic stenosis.

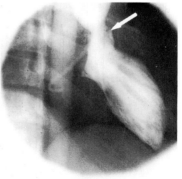

Fig. 86 LV angiogram showing supravalvar aortic stenosis.

Aortic stenosis (2)

Investigations

Electrocardiography. 85% of patients with significant aortic stenosis have voltage criteria of LVH (maximum S wave V_{1-3} + maximum R wave V_{4-6} > 35 mm with standard ECG calibration). ST depression and T wave inversion may develop over the lateral chest leads (V_4–V_6) referred to as a *strain* pattern. Old anterior myocardial infarction may be diagnosed inappropriately because of poor anterior R wave progression. In rare patients fibrocalcific encroachment on the atrioventricular node may lead to heart block.

Chest X-ray. The heart size is typically normal although a *bulky* appearance may be suggested. The ascending aorta may be dilated proximally (post-stenotic dilatation). Valve calcification is best appreciated on the lateral chest film and its absence in a patient over 35 years of age has been said to exclude significant aortic stenosis.

Echocardiography. Diagnostic investigation. Demonstrates the anatomy of the valve indicating the extent of disruption of normal architecture. Doppler study allows the measurement of the gradient across the valve giving an objective index of severity. LVH is demonstrated and ventricular function may also be assessed. Some patients at low risk of coronary artery disease (young, non-smokers) may proceed to valve replacement without cardiac catheterization.

Cardiac catheterization. Indicated in patients at risk of coronary artery disease in whom coronary surgery at the time of aortic valve replacement may be needed.

Natural history

Aortic stenosis typically progresses slowly and remains asymptomatic for many years. Asymptomatic individuals with mild to moderate stenosis require follow-up to detect evidence of progression. Valve replacement is indicated in all patients who develop symptoms and should not be delayed until irreversible ventricular damage has occurred. Aortic valvotomy (open surgery or transvenous balloon valvotomy) may be possible in young patients with congenital disease.

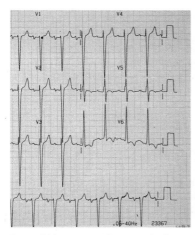

Fig. 87 ECG showing LV hypertrophy from patient with aortic stenosis.

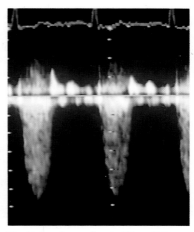

Fig. 88 Doppler gradient (>100 mmHg) across stenotic valve.

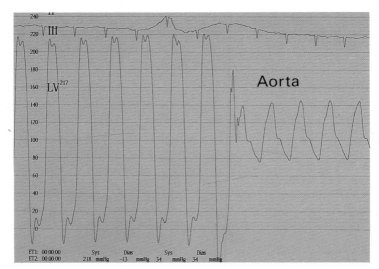

Fig. 89 'Pull-back' gradient from LV to aorta of 80 mmHg measured as catheter withdrawn across aortic valve in patient with severe AS.

Aortic stenosis (3)

Valve replacement

The significant advance in the management of patients with valve disease has been valve replacement. Valve replacement is performed via a median sternotomy on cardiopulmonary bypass. The heart is arrested using cardioplegia and the operation carried out under hypothermia. The valve to be replaced is excised and the annulus measured, the prosthetic valve is inserted and sutured into place. Hospital mortality is usually of the order of 1–4% for elective valve replacement.

Choice of valve prosthesis

Two main types of prosthetic valve are available:

1. Mechanical valves   e.g. St. Jude bi-leaflet disc, Björk-Shiley tilting disc and Starr–Edwards caged ball device. Constitute more than 85% valves used.

2. Tissue valves   e.g. pig valves, cryo-preserved homograft, bovine pericardium. In general, mechanical valves are resilient with a low failure rate but are thrombogenic and require lifelong anticoagulation. Tissue valves have a limited lifespan and need replacement usually after 8–12 years; however they may be used without anticoagulants and are used in patients with special risks, e.g. the elderly.

Problems with prosthetic valves

Endocarditis: patients with prosthetic valves need to follow approved antibiotic prophylaxis regimes.

Embolism: most dramatic manifestation is cerebral embolism but other vascular beds can be involved.

Thrombosis   is relatively uncommon but can follow discontinuation of anticoagulants. Dull thuds rather than clear clicks are heard on auscultation and immediate surgery is usually indicated; thrombolysis has been used in selected patients.

Bleeding: the risk of warfarin.

Prosthetic failure: *Mechanical*—unusual (<0.1% per annum) but catastrophic presenting with cardiogenic shock and no audible clicks—needs immediate surgery. *Tissue-valve failure* is less dramatic with progressive stenosis or regurgitation leading to heart failure.

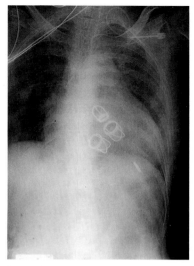

Fig. 90 Chest X-ray of three valves in situ.

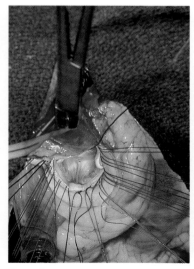

Fig. 91 Valve replacement (the operation).

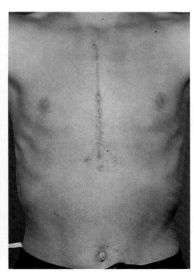

Fig. 92 Median sternotomy.

13 / Aortic regurgitation

Aetiology

Results either from defect of valve leaflets or from aortic root dilatation. Rheumatic disease and syphilis are now rare causes with infective endocarditis and idiopathic root dilatation being relatively more common.

Valvular. Causes include bicuspid aortic valve (approximately 25%), infective endocarditis, myxomatous degeneration (floppy aortic valve), rheumatic heart disease (<10%) and trauma.

Root. Annulo-aortic ectasia, cystic medio-necrosis (isolated or as part of a Marfan syndrome), osteogenesis imperfecta, syphilis and inflammatory diseases including ankylosing spondylitis, Reiter syndrome and ulcerative colitis are all causes. Aortic dissection may present with acute aortic regurgitation.

Symptoms

Initial symptoms in patients with chronic aortic regurgitation often relate to augmented stroke volume with complaints of a forceful heart beat and pulsations in the neck. Symptoms of heart failure ensue as the left ventricle fails. Patients with acute aortic regurgitation, e.g. infective endocarditis, may have a very abrupt onset of left heart failure with vascular collapse.

Signs

With moderate to severe chronic aortic regurgitation the peripheral signs of augmented forward stroke volume are usually well marked, e.g. visible pulsations in the neck (Corrigan's sign). The pulse is collapsing in quality (*waterhammer pulse*). The apex beat is displaced due to left ventricular dilatation and is hyperdynamic (exaggerated normal) in quality. The early diastolic murmur is heard best at the lower left sternal edge with the patient sitting up holding their breath in expiration. In patients with acute aortic regurgitation the clinical signs are not usually so impressive. The diagnosis needs careful consideration in any patient presenting with unexplained acute heart failure.

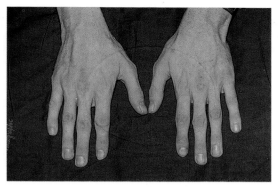

Fig. 93 Arachnodactyly (Marfan syndrome).

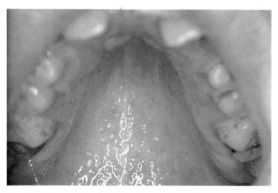

Fig. 94 High-arched palate (Marfan syndrome).

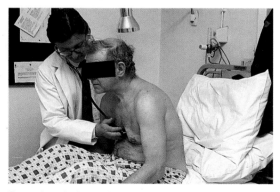

Fig. 95 Auscultation: early diastolic murmur (patient in expiration).

Aortic regurgitation (2)

Investigations

Chest X-ray. Dilatation of the aortic root is usual. Left ventricular dilatation is also present and may be marked. Cardiac enlargement is not usually a feature of acute aortic regurgitation where pulmonary oedema is more commonly seen.

ECG. LVH is usual with chronic aortic regurgitation but is not a feature of acute regurgitation.

Echocardiography. Two-dimensional echocardiography is often useful in identifying the cause of aortic regurgitation; it may show aortic root dilatation, valvular vegetations or a bicuspid valve. Doppler studies are a sensitive indicator of aortic regurgitation and can provide an index of the severity of the disease. Echocardiography allows serial assessment of left ventricular function. Increased left ventricular systolic dimensions are an indicator of impending irreversible dysfunction.

Aortography. Classical method for defining the severity of aortic regurgitation. Dye injected into the aortic root refluxes into the left ventricle, with the volume and delay in clearance indicating the severity of regurgitation.

Natural history

Chronic aortic regurgitation is characterized by an extended asymptomatic period where compensation is maintained by dilatation and hypertrophy of the left ventricle. During this phase the ejection fraction will often remain normal. Ultimately LVH and failure supervene and correct timing of valve replacement is therefore critical.

Management

Any symptomatic patient with aortic regurgitation should undergo investigation with a view to aortic valve replacement. Patients with asymptomatic aortic regurgitation may benefit from vasodilators, and valve replacement may be indicated if there are signs of left ventricular dysfunction. However, the optimal timing of surgery in these patients is uncertain.

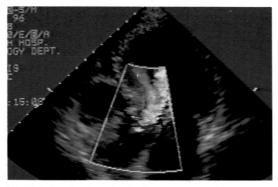

Fig. 96 Colour flow Doppler showing regurgitant jet in diastole.

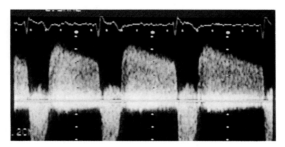

Fig. 97 Continuous wave Doppler in mixed aortic valve disease.

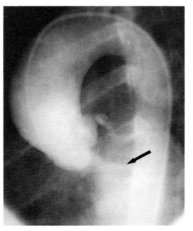

Fig. 98 Aortogram with dilatation of the
aortic root and aortic regurgitation.

Aetiology

1. Coronary artery disease. Patients with coronary artery disease usually develop mitral regurgitation as a consequence of left ventricular dilatation causing stretching of the valve ring or ischaemia causing papillary muscle dysfunction.

2. Mitral prolapse (see below).

3. Mitral annular calcification. Important cause of mitral regurgitation in elderly patients occurring secondary to the deposition of calcium in the basal portions of the mitral leaflets. Mitral regurgitation may also develop in patients with cardiomyopathy, rheumatic heart disease (usually associated with mitral stenosis), systemic lupus erythematosus (Libman–Sacks endocarditis), Marfan syndrome, osteogenesis imperfecta and following valve destruction in endocarditis. Congenital mitral regurgitation may accompany atrial septal defects or atrioventricular septal defects.

Clinical picture

The symptoms are usually those of heart failure with dyspnoea and lethargy. The characteristic finding on examination is a pansystolic murmur loudest at the apex with radiation to the axilla but often heard throughout the precordium. With increasing severity there is a left ventricular gallop (S3), diastolic flow murmur and systolic thrill.

Investigations

Chest X-ray. Cardiomegaly is usually present with specifically left atrial and left ventricular enlargement. Calcification of the mitral annulus may be seen. Pulmonary congestion and oedema may be present.

Electrocardiography. LVH is often present. In the patient remaining in sinus rhythm evidence of left atrial enlargement may be seen (P mitrale); atrial fibrillation however is common. The ECG may provide a clue to aetiology, e.g. Q waves indicating prior myocardial infarction.

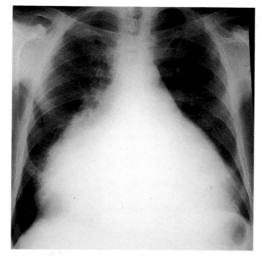

Fig. 99 'Cor-bovinum': massive cardiomegaly.

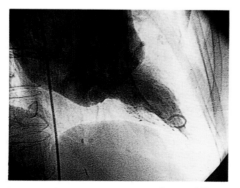

Fig. 100 Left ventricular angiogram of severe MR.

Mitral regurgitation (2)

Investigations (cont.)

Echocardiography. Two-dimensional echocardiography demonstrates an enlarged left atrium and hyperdynamic left ventricle in most patients. The aetiology may be apparent from other features, e.g. a *rheumatic* valve, submitral calcification, chordal rupture, vegetations, regional wall motion abnormality or flail mitral leaflets. Doppler interrogation shows a high velocity jet in the left atrium visible in systole.

Cardiac catheterization. Left atrial pressure (pulmonary capillary wedge pressure) is usually elevated with a large regurgitant systolic *v* wave. Left ventriculography demonstrates reflux from the left ventricle to the left atrium during systole. The rate and extent of opacification is used as an index of the severity of regurgitation.

Natural history

The natural history of mitral regurgitation is variable and dependent on the underlying cause. Timing of operation is controversial. Long-standing mitral regurgitation may lead to impairment of left ventricular function which is not reversed by mitral valve surgery. Therefore asymptomatic patients with severe mitral regurgitation may need surgery.

Surgery

Valve repair with the insertion of a prosthetic annular ring but preservation of the integral valve structure is increasingly used, though it is not suitable for some patients who still require mitral valve replacement.

Mitral valve prolapse

An increasingly diagnosed valve lesion. Incidence dependent on the criteria applied but ranges of 3–15% are quoted for otherwise normal women. Patients are usually symptom-free but may complain of atypical chest pain and palpitations. A spectrum of disease exists from mild prolapse (click only) through mild mitral regurgitation (click + late systolic murmur) to severe mitral regurgitation (pansystolic murmur). Severe mitral regurgitation occurs in older males and requires valve surgery. Definitive diagnosis relies on echocardiography which demonstrates mitral leaflet prolapse in systole. Patients with murmurs require antibiotic prophylaxis against endocarditis.

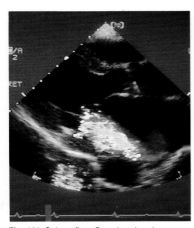

Fig. 101 Colour flow Doppler showing regurgitant jet across the mitral valve from LV to left atrium.

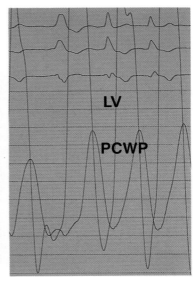

Fig. 102 Large 'v' wave in pulmonary capillary wedge pressure trace (simultaneous LV and PCWP trace).

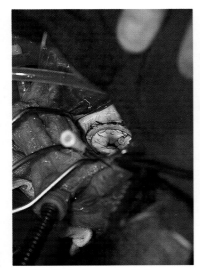

Fig. 103 Mitral valve repair with the insertion of prosthetic 'Carpentier' ring.

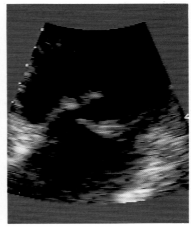

Fig. 104 Two-dimensional echocardiogram: prolapse of the posterior mitral valve leaflet.

Aetiology

The incidence of rheumatic fever has fallen sharply in the Western world, but most patients with mitral stenosis have had rheumatic carditis in the past. This results in contraction, scarring and fusion of the valve leaflets and shortening and fusion of the chordae tendiniae over time. Rare patients have congenital mitral stenosis usually in conjunction with other anomalies. Systemic lupus erythematosus particularly when associated with circulating antiphospholipid antibodies is a recognized albeit rare cause.

Symptoms

Symptoms are those of pulmonary venous congestion with dyspnoea, orthopnoea and paroxysmal nocturnal dyspnoea. Pulmonary hypertension leads to right ventricular dilatation and failure with peripheral oedema and abdominal swelling. Some patients present with systemic embolism from clot arising in the left atrium. Prior to the introduction of surgery and the use of anticoagulants, >25% of deaths were from this cause.

Signs

Patients with mitral stenosis may have the mitral facies but this appearance lacks specificity. Atrial fibrillation is very common and indeed usual with moderate to severe disease. The characteristic findings in mitral stenosis are on auscultation. With a mobile valve the first heart sound is loud and often palpable (*tapping* apex) and an opening snap is present. A low-pitched diastolic rumbling murmur is heard most easily at the apex with the patient in the left lateral position. Loss of valve pliability due to calcification is usually accompanied by a loss of the opening snap and muffling of the first heart sound. An atrial myxoma may produce similar clinical signs.

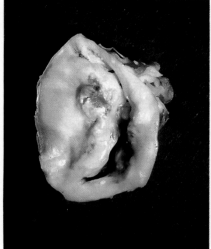

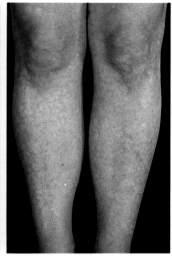

Fig. 105 Mitral stenosis with a 'fish mouth' orifice.

Fig. 106 Livedo reticularis in the antiphospholipid syndrome.

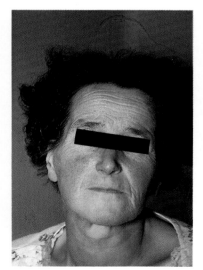

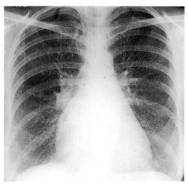

Fig. 108 Typical chest X-ray in mitral stenosis, showing straight left heart border.

Fig. 107 Mitral facies.

Mitral stenosis (2)

Investigations

Chest X-ray. Demonstrates enlargement of the left atrium and right ventricle. Pulmonary blood flow is usually redistributed to the upper lobes and Kerley B lines develop. Chronic pulmonary interstitial oedema may lead to pulmonary haemosiderosis and ossification with small islands of bone visible as dense nodules in the lung fields.

Electrocardiogram. Most patients are in atrial fibrillation. Patients in sinus rhythm show evidence of left atrial enlargement (P mitrale). Pulmonary hypertension leads to right axis deviation.

Echocardiography. Two-dimensional echocardiography shows a deformed mitral apparatus with doming of the mitral valve. Using two-dimensional echo the mitral valve area may be directly planimetered. Doppler echo can assess the gradient across the valve and estimate valve area.

Cardiac catheterization. A pressure gradient is present between the left atrial (pulmonary capillary wedge pressure) and left ventricular pressure during diastole and allows calculation of the valve area.

Natural history

Symptoms do not usually develop for 20 years after rheumatic carditis with slow development thereafter.

Management

Medical. All patients with mitral stenosis and atrial fibrillation require anticoagulation to reduce the risk of systemic embolism. Digoxin is usually required for patients with atrial fibrillation to control the ventricular response and diuretics may also be needed.

Interventional. Indicated in symptomatic patients. *Transvenous balloon valvuloplasty.* The treatment of choice in most patients; even non-pliable calcified valves can be successfully dilated. The technique requires puncture of the inter-atrial septum and inflation across the valve of an Inoue balloon.

Mitral valve surgery. Open mitral valvotomy or mitral valve replacement are now needed less frequently in patients with pure mitral stenosis.

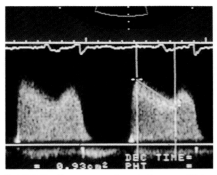

Fig. 109 Continuous wave Doppler in severe MS with valve area of 0.93 cm².

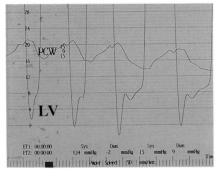

Fig. 110 Transvalvar gradient demonstrated between the LV and PWP at right and left heart catheterization.

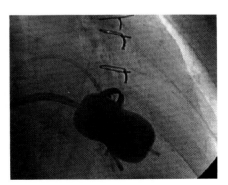

Fig. 111 Mitral valvuloplasty using the 'Inoue' balloon.

16 / Infective endocarditis

Definition

Infective endocarditis usually refers to bacterial infection of the heart valves. Infection with fungi (e.g. candida), chlamydiae or rickettsiae also occur although less frequently. Terms such as *acute* and *subacute bacterial endocarditis* (SBE) are now used less.

Risk factors

Approximately 3000–4000 cases occur annually in the United Kingdom and the figure may be increasing. Any patient with damage to the endocardium is at increased risk of infective endocarditis. Those with valvular heart disease especially non-rheumatic (bicuspid aortic valves, mitral valve prolapse) and patients with congenital heart disease (e.g. ventricular septal defect, patent ductus arteriosus but not atrial septal defect) constitute the traditional high-risk groups. New risk groups have become prominent and include intravenous drug abusers (right-sided endocarditis more common) and those with prosthetic heart valves. Patients at risk should maintain good dental hygiene and receive antibiotic prophylaxis for dental and surgical procedures.

Microbiology

A wide range of organisms can cause infective endocarditis. The most common are viridans streptococci—normal mouth flora whose surface glycoproteins enhance adherence to heart valves. Specific risk groups are prone to particular infections, e.g. the elderly to group D streptococci and intravenous drug addicts to *Staphylococcus spp.*

Pathology

Blood-borne organisms become lodged with platelets at the site of endocardial damage with the subsequent development of vegetations. These can grow quite large particularly following infection with, for example, *Staphylococcus aureus* and fungi. Invasion into neighbouring structures can lead to valve incompetence, conduction defects and abscess formation.

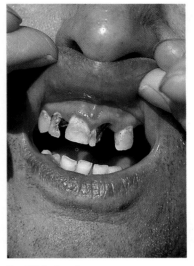

Fig. 112 Bad teeth.

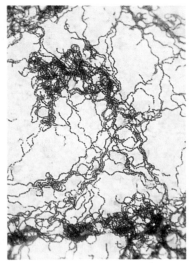

Fig. 113 *Streptococcus viridans.*

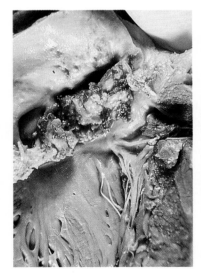

Fig. 114 Postmortem pathology of the aortic valve showing extensive vegetations.

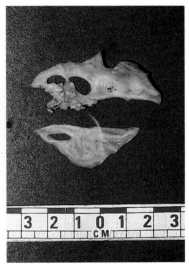

Fig. 115 Vegetations demonstrated clearly on aortic valve after removal at valve replacement.

Infective endocarditis (2)

Clinical recognition

Early diagnosis is the key to successful management. Relevant features include antecedent cardiac disease, recent dental or surgical procedures or a history of intravenous drug abuse. The diagnosis should be considered in any patient with unexplained fever, rashes, anaemia, murmurs or heart failure. A range of peripheral stigmata are described which may be relatively specific, e.g. Osler's nodes, Janeway lesions, or non-specific, e.g. clubbing, petechiae, leucocytoclastic vasculitis or splinter haemorrhages.

Investigations

Blood cultures.   If the diagnosis is a possibility then a series of blood cultures should be obtained and only then should intravenous antibiotics be commenced. The results of microbiology should not be awaited if there is reasonable clinical suspicion as it introduces unnecessary delay.

Electrocardiography.   The ECG is important as conduction disturbances suggest extension of the infection into neighbouring myocardium.

Urine examination.   Infective endocarditis may be complicated by renal involvement (usually glomerulonephritis) and urine microscopy is indicated in all patients.

Echocardiography.   Trans-thoracic echo allows visualization of vegetations ≥ 3 mm diameter. Transoesophageal echo is more sensitive and is the imaging modality of choice for prosthetic valve endocarditis and for aortic root abscess formation.

Management

Mortality from infective endocarditis remains high at approximately 20%. The choice of antibiotic and the duration of therapy should be decided in consultation with microbiologists. Intravenous therapy with antibiotics given in hospital remains standard practice. All patients should be reviewed by a cardiologist at an early stage; valve surgery is indicated if there is haemodynamic deterioration, persistent infection, abscess formation, fungal or Staph. aureus infection, systemic emboli or large mobile vegetations.

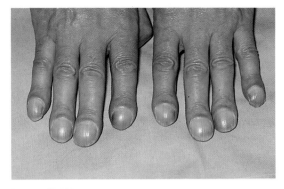

Fig. 116 Clubbing.

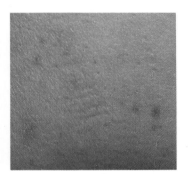

Fig. 117 Petechiae.

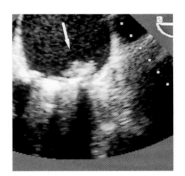

Fig. 118 Large vegetation on a mitral valve prosthesis.

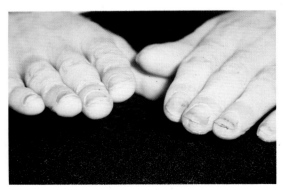

Fig. 119 Extensive splinter haemorrhages.

Acute pericarditis

Inflammation of the pericardium is most commonly due to infection with viruses, e.g. Coxsackie B, Echo 8, mumps, influenza and Epstein Barr. However, the range of causes is widespread and includes bacteria, rheumatic diseases, neoplasms, uraemia and myocardial infarction.

The clinical syndrome is characterized by chest pain (retrosternal, radiating to the arms and shoulders and typically eased by sitting forward) and a pericardial friction rub. Serial repolarization changes on the ECG occur in 90% of cases. ST elevation on the ECG is usually present in many leads and is concave upwards which serves to distinguish it from the ST changes of acute myocardial infarction. PR segment depression is pathognomonic. The CXR is often normal but echocardiography may reveal a small pericardial effusion. Management is symptomatic with anti-inflammatory analgesics and bedrest as the disease is self-limiting in most patients.

Pericardial effusion

The development of an effusion in the pericardial space may occur with inflammation of the pericardium. The effusion is often asymptomatic but large effusions with cardiac compression lead to cardiac tamponade (hypotension, pulsus paradoxus and an elevated JVP). On the chest X-ray the cardiac silhouette does not usually widen until >250 ml fluid has accumulated. With a large effusion a globular appearance is characteristic. Echocardiography provides the diagnosis and allows planning of therapy. Pericardiocentesis is required to relieve haemodynamically significant effusions and obtain material for diagnosis. Chronic pericardial effusions may require open surgical drainage, the creation of a pericardial window and in some cases pericardectomy.

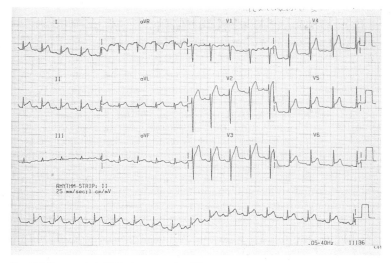

Fig. 120 Characteristic ECG of acute pericarditis.

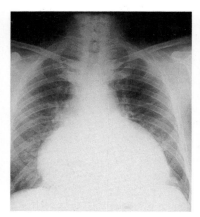

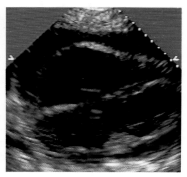

Fig. 122 Two-dimensional echocardiogram showing pericardial effusion.

Fig. 121 Chest X-ray in patient with large pericardial effusion.

18 / Constrictive pericarditis

Definition

Constrictive pericarditis arises when a rigid inelastic pericardium adheres to the heart resulting in impairment of diastolic filling. The diagnosis is often missed or delayed but is particularly important, as surgical débridement of the pericardium results in cure. Tuberculosis remains a common cause of constrictive pericarditis world-wide although it is an infrequent cause (<10%) in developed countries. Most cases now arise following previous cardiac surgery or mediastinal radiation although rheumatoid disease, previous viral infection or trauma can also result in pericardial constriction. Many cases remain idiopathic.

Clinical picture

Symptoms are usually those of heart failure with dyspnoea and oedema. Abdominal swelling with hepatomegaly and ascites more marked than peripheral oedema may lead to a mistaken diagnosis of liver disease. The key clinical signs are of a raised jugular venous pressure persisting despite diuretic therapy and an early 3rd heart sound (pericardial knock) on auscultation.

Investigations

Pericardial calcification on a lateral CXR is a useful clue but is not diagnostic of constriction. Findings on echocardiography are in general non-specific. The differential diagnosis from restrictive cardiomyopathy can be difficult since similar haemodynamic derangements are produced. Differentiation depends on endomyocardial biopsy (perhaps showing amyloid infiltration) or on CT scan or Magnetic Resonance Imaging (showing thickened pericardium).

Management

Patients with constrictive pericarditis benefit from complete surgical resection of the pericardium usually carried out under cardiopulmonary bypass. Operative mortality is however still as high as 5–10% in most centres.

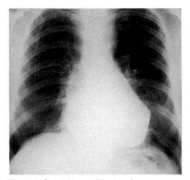

Fig. 123 Chest X-ray: PA showing pericardial calcification.

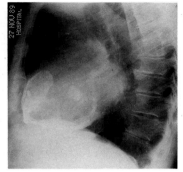

Fig. 124 Chest X-ray: lateral showing pericardial calcification.

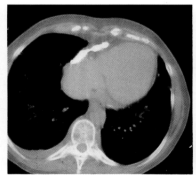

Fig. 125 CT scan: transverse cut showing localized pericardial calcification.

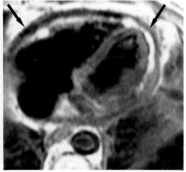

Fig. 126 MRI scan: transverse cut showing thickened pericardium as signal void.

The spectrum of abnormalities of cardiac rhythm ranges from benign, clinically insignificant, disturbances of normal conduction to life-threatening arrhythmias. On a single ambulatory ECG recording more than 50% of normal individuals will have premature beats; at the dangerous end of the spectrum 50 Americans die every hour of malignant ventricular arrhythmia.

Premature beats (extrasystoles)

Definition

Cardiac contractions initiated by premature ectopic foci. The ventricles are the most common site of origin but they may also arise from the atria, junctional zone or, rarely, the sinus node.

Clinical picture

Premature beats are one of the most common causes of palpitation with the heart beat being described as *turning over* or *skipping a beat*. They are usually noted at night or when the patient is otherwise at rest. The diagnosis may be suggested on the 12-lead ECG at the initial consultation (present on 1% of standard ECGs) but may need ambulatory electrocardiography.

Significance

Infrequent ventricular premature beats occurring in the absence of underlying heart disease are normal. Following myocardial infarction or, in patients with structural heart disease frequent (>10 per h), complex premature ventricular beats are a bad prognostic sign. In these patients they probably serve principally as a marker of the severity of the underlying disorder, and their suppression does not improve prognosis.

Management

The majority of patients need reassurance. Very symptomatic patients may benefit from drug therapy, beta-blockers being successful in many. In patients with symptomatic premature beats and underlying heart disease, the potentially serious side-effects of drug therapy such as proarrhythmia should be weighed against the ill-defined benefits.

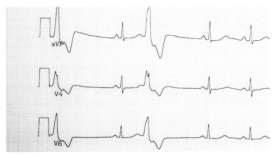

Fig. 127 Ventricular ectopy.

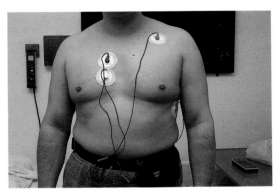

Fig. 128 Patient wearing Holter monitor.

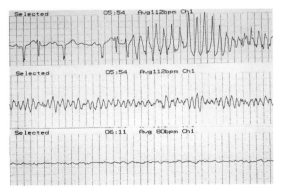

Fig. 129 Sinus rhythm leading to polymorphic VT, VF and asystole on ambulatory tape.

Incidence

Atrial fibrillation (AF) is a very common arrhythmia affecting 2–5% of the population >60 years of age, but may also affect younger patients.

Definition

Characterized by rapid disorganized atrial depolarization at rates exceeding 300/min with an irregular ventricular response often at rates greater than 120/min. The main consequences are decreased cardiac efficiency and an increased incidence of stroke.

Aetiology

Most patients with atrial fibrillation have underlying structural heart disease, e.g. coronary artery disease, rheumatic heart disease, hypertensive heart disease or chronic heart failure. Thyrotoxicosis should be considered as a cause in any patient even in the absence of other evidence of the disease. Other causes include infection, particularly pneumonia, pulmonary embolism and alcohol. Patients with no apparent cause following a careful history and exclusion of structural heart disease are said to have *lone* atrial fibrillation.

Symptoms

Irregular palpitations, dizziness and breathlessness are common symptoms. In patients with structural heart disease, a rapid ventricular response may lead to decreased cardiac efficiency with a fall in cardiac output and symptoms of pulmonary congestion. Patients may present with an acute onset or an established arrhythmia with non-specific symptoms. Some patients have paroxysmal atrial fibrillation suggested initially by a clinical history of intermittent fast irregular palpitations and confirmed using ambulatory electrocardiography.

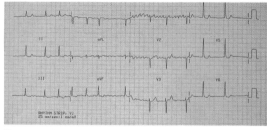

Fig. 130 ECG showing 'coarse' (clearly defined 'f' waves) atrial fibrillation.

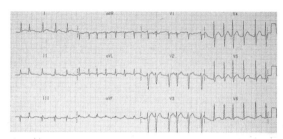

Fig. 131 ECG showing 'fine' atrial fibrillation.

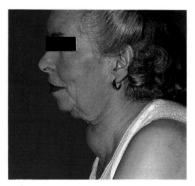

Fig. 132 Thyrotoxic goitre.

Atrial fibrillation (2)

Investigations

All patients presenting with atrial fibrillation require a number of baseline investigations.

Electrocardiography. Although a presumptive diagnosis of atrial fibrillation can often be made clinically the diagnosis is of such importance that an ECG should be obtained in all cases.

Thyroid function tests. Essential in all patients even with no other evidence of thyroid overactivity.

Echocardiography. Essential in all patients with atrial fibrillation. It is important to exclude underlying valvular heart disease, assess left ventricular function and left atrial size and look for evidence of thrombus.

Complications

The main complications, e.g. stroke, arise from systemic embolism, although the emboli may originate from the great vessels rather than from the heart. Overall the risk of stroke in atrial fibrillation is 5 times that of age-matched controls. 20% of all strokes occur in patients with non-valvular atrial fibrillation.

Management

Acute AF. DC cardioversion is the treatment of choice in the haemodynamically compromised patient with fast AF. Antiarrhythmic drugs may be used to achieve *chemical cardioversion* in stable patients. Patients with paroxysmal atrial fibrillation (PAF) may benefit from drug prophylaxis with amiodarone, sotalol, quinidine etc.

Chronic AF: *1. Control of ventricular rate.* Digoxin is commonly used but control of ventricular rate on exercise is often inadequate. Other atrioventricular nodal blocking drugs can be added if necessary. Non-pharmacological treatment includes catheter ablation of the AV node or atrial tissue, and surgical division of the atria (e.g. MAZE operation). *2. Protection against systemic embolism.* All patients with atrial fibrillation due to rheumatic disease should receive warfarin. Patients with non-rheumatic atrial fibrillation with or without structural heart disease should also be considered for anticoagulation. Careful individualization of warfarin therapy reduces the risk of adverse effects from bleeding, but some side-effects such as skin necrosis are idiosyncratic.

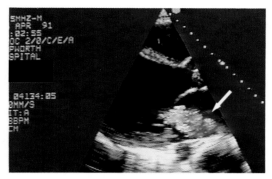

Fig. 133 Colour flow Doppler showing severe mitral regurgitation in a patient presenting with AF.

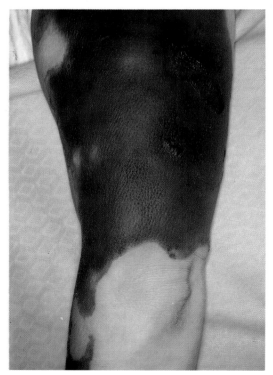

Fig. 134 Skin necrosis in patient with protein C deficiency given warfarin.

Atrial flutter

Less common than atrial fibrillation. The atrial rate of depolarization is often around 300 beats/min but 2 : 1 atrioventricular block is often present, giving ventricular rates of around 150 bpm. Electrocardiography reveals the classic *saw tooth* appearance of atrial activity. Palpitations, dizziness and breathlessness are common symptoms. Syncope may occur if 1 : 1 conduction with a ventricular rate of 300/min occurs. In patients with coronary disease, angina or symptoms of heart failure may supervene. Atrial flutter is five times more common in men than women, and may be associated with lung disease, valve disease, thyrotoxicosis, or follow heart surgery.

Management

Acute treatment. DC cardioversion is usually the treatment of choice. Sinus rhythm is restored in nearly all patients.

Long-term treatment. Repeated paroxysms may be controlled with antiarrhythmic agents. Catheter ablation using radiofrequency energy is successful in selected patients. For patients with established, chronic atrial flutter, ventricular rate control with drugs that slow AV node conduction may be sufficient. The risk of thromboembolism appears to be lower than that with AF, but patients with structural heart disease should be considered for anticoagulation.

Atrial tachycardia

A less common atrial arrhythmia (ventricular rate normally 120–220 bpm), with unifocal or multifocal forms. Non-sustained episodes may occur in normal subjects, but patients with sustained episodes usually have underlying heart disease. Incessant atrial tachycardia in childhood may lead to a dilated cardiomyopathy. Symptomatic patients may benefit from antiarrhythmic drug treatment, catheter or surgical ablation.

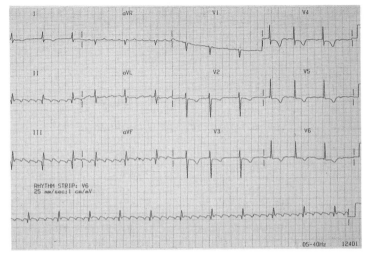

Fig. 135 Classic 'saw-tooth' appearance of ECG in atrial flutter.

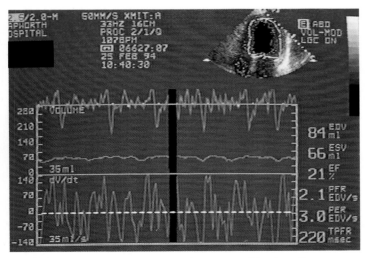

Fig. 136 Tachycardiomyopathy in patient with *incessant* atrial tachycardia.

These arrhythmias may present at any age including childhood and usually occur in otherwise functionally normal hearts. Approximately half of patients have *atrioventricular nodal re-entrant tachycardia* (AVNRT) with a circus movement of depolarization in the atrioventricular nodal (junctional) region producing a regular narrow complex tachycardia. Re-entry may also occur via accessory atrioventricular pathways giving rise to *atrioventricular re-entrant tachycardia* (AVRT), as in the pre-excitation syndromes (e.g. Wolff–Parkinson–White) and in patients with *concealed* accessory pathways.

Symptoms

A history of the sudden onset of rapid regular palpitations lasting from minutes to hours is characteristic. Vagotonic manoeuvres (e.g. Valsalva) may have been identified by the patient as being helpful in terminating symptoms. Dizziness, anxiety and breathlessness are relatively mild and only occasionally severe and incapacitating in patients with otherwise normal hearts. In patients with other cardiac disease angina, heart failure or syncope may be precipitated.

Diagnosis

The 12-lead ECG in AVNRT is usually normal during sinus rhythm. Establishing the diagnosis requires an ECG recorded during an attack (12-lead ECG or obtained using ambulatory electrocardiography); this usually shows a narrow complex tachycardia with a rate of 160–250 bpm. In patients with infrequent attacks a patient-activated recording device may be necessary. The diagnosis is often apparent from examining the pattern of atrial activity on the 12-lead ECG but precise diagnosis requires an electrophysiological study (EPS). Radiofrequency ablation can be performed at the same sitting.

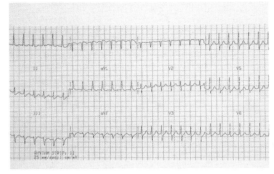

Fig. 137 ECG in patient with AVNRT.

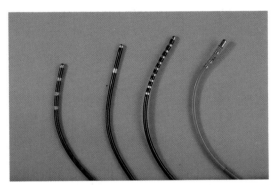

Fig. 138 Intracardiac pacing leads used for electrophysiological studies.

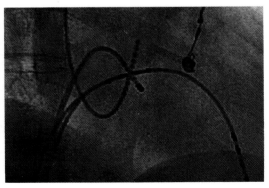

Fig. 139 Leads positioned for an electrophysiological study.

Junctional arrhythmias (2)

1. Termination. Arrhythmia termination may be attempted using vagotonic manoeuvres, e.g. Valsalva manoeuvre or carotid sinus massage, but these are usually unsuccessful in those patients presenting to hospital. Drug termination should be attempted in the first instance using intravenous adenosine. Supraventricular arrhythmias with aberrant conduction (wide QRS complex) are for the purposes of immediate therapy best regarded as rare and treatment should be as for ventricular tachycardia unless the diagnosis is certain.

2. Prophylaxis. Drug therapy is often tried for prophylaxis in patients with frequent disabling episodes of arrhythmia but adequate symptom suppression may prove difficult.

3. Cure. Patients remaining symptomatic on drug therapy usually benefit from catheter ablation of accessory atrioventricular connections using radiofrequency energy.

Pre-excitation syndromes
Pre-excitation is defined as early depolarization of ventricular myocardium via an alternative route bypassing the atrioventricular node. The Wolff–Parkinson–White (WPW) syndrome is the most common form, characterized anatomically by an accessory connection(s) between atria and ventricle. Patients usually present with palpitations. The eponym refers to the ECG appearances in conjunction with symptoms; the incidence is unknown but the ECG abnormality is present in 0.3% of routine recordings. The 12-lead ECG in sinus rhythm shows a short PR interval and a delta wave (slurred onset of the QRS leading to wide complex). Symptomatic patients not responding to drug therapy require radiofrequency catheter ablation of the accessory pathway.

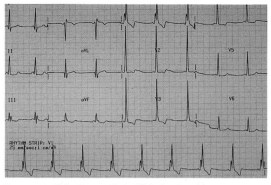

Fig. 140 Wolff–Parkinson–White ECG showing delta waves.

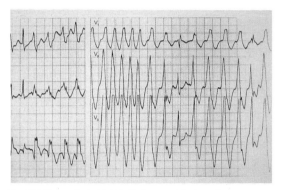

Fig. 141 Pre-excited atrial fibrillation: ventricular rate >300 bpm.

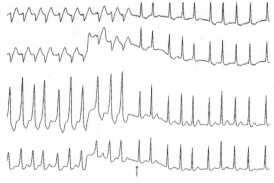

Fig. 142 Radiofrequency ablation in WPW: following ablation the delta wave disappears.

Definitions

Five or more ventricular premature beats occurring consecutively define ventricular tachycardia. Non-sustained ventricular tachycardia terminates spontaneously in <30 s. Sustained ventricular tachycardia lasts >30 s or requires cardioversion to terminate the arrhythmia because of haemodynamic collapse.

Aetiology

Coronary artery disease. Most patients with ventricular tachycardia have underlying coronary artery disease and previous myocardial infarction.

Cardiomyopathy. Dilated and hypertrophic cardiomyopathy predispose to ventricular tachycardia which contributes to increased risk of sudden death. Other causes include the congenital long QT syndromes, some drug-induced arrhythmias (*torsade de pointes*), and arrhythmogenic right ventricular dysplasia (ARVD). In some patients with *structurally normal hearts* the site of origin is in the right ventricular outflow tract or the Purkinje fascicles and may be amenable to ablative therapy.

Presentation

Ventricular tachycardia may be asymptomatic or present with bouts of palpitations, dyspnoea or chest pain; more dramatic presentations with syncope are also common. Ventricular tachycardia is a bad prognostic marker in patients with coronary disease.

Diagnosis

In patients presenting with tachycardia the diagnosis is usually apparent from the 12-lead ECG. Ventricular tachycardia is a *broad complex tachycardia* and is by far the most common cause of this ECG pattern in older patients. Despite this, it continues to be confused with supraventricular tachycardia with aberrant conduction. The principal ECG features that distinguish ventricular tachycardia from aberrantly conducted supraventricular arrhythmia are atrioventricular dissociation, very broad QRS complexes (>140 ms) and marked axis deviation. (e.g. positive QRS complex in aVR).

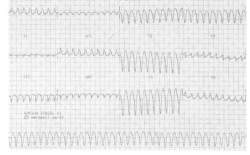

Fig. 143 Ventricular tachycardia.

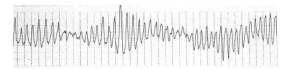

Fig. 144 Polymorphic ventricular tachycardia.

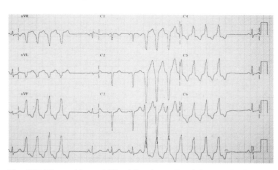

Fig. 145 'Normal heart VT' arising from the right ventricular outflow tract.

Ventricular tachycardia (2)

Investigations

Patients with ventricular tachycardia are at increased risk of sudden cardiac death (SCD) and require thorough investigation.

General. Echocardiography, stress testing and coronary arteriography, and measurement of ejection fraction are usually required in all patients.

Electrophysiological investigation. Patients presenting with sustained ventricular tachycardia or following resuscitation from sudden cardiac death should be reviewed by a cardiologist with a view to electrophysiological studies.

Management

Management is complex and evolving and best undertaken by specialist cardiac electrophysiologists.

Pharmacological. Empirical drug therapy other than beta-blockers or amiodarone is generally not recommended. Drug therapy determined by serial electrophysiologic testing is preferable, but the incidence of sudden cardiac death is still significant in patients with pharmacologically *suppressed* arrhythmias. Amiodarone is the most effective antiarrhythmic drug, but is complicated by side-effects, the most serious of which is pulmonary fibrosis.

Device therapy. In recent years there has been a great increase in the use of implanted devices to terminate ventricular tachycardia. Implantable cardioverter defibrillators (ICDs) recognize the arrhythmia and then terminate that arrhythmia usually by pacing or by the delivery of a defibrillating shock. These devices can be placed with transvenous leads and their use is likely to increase. In most countries this may be constrained by the significant financial costs.

Curative therapy. Selected patients benefit from electrophysiologically guided surgery to remove the arrhythmogenic substrate, with or without revascularization. Transvenous catheter ablation may also prove useful in selected patients, particularly in those with either *normal heart VT* or an *incessant* ventricular arrhythmia.

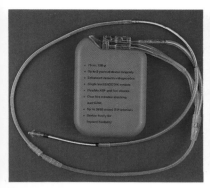

Fig. 146 Implantable cardioverter defibrillator.

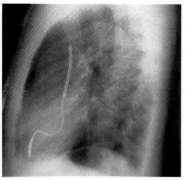

Fig. 147 Lateral chest X-ray showing implantable defibrillator lead in right ventricle.

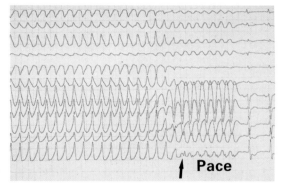

Fig. 148 Overdrive pacing of VT to sinus rhythm.

Sudden cardiac death (SCD) is defined as death within 1 h of acute symptoms and is the mode of death in 50% of patients who die with heart disease, being responsible for 300 000 deaths a year in the United States. Availability of effective and more widespread resuscitation has led to the concept of *reversible* death.

Aetiology

Coronary disease is the most common underlying structural heart defect, responsible for 65% of sudden death in men and 40% of women. Patients with a low ejection fraction, history of heart failure, and survivors of a cardiac arrest are at particular risk. LVH is a common finding and an independent risk factor for SCD. Hypertrophic or dilated cardiomyopathy are found in 2–3% of patients.

Mechanism

Ventricular tachycardia or fibrillation is estimated to be the cause in 80% of cases; bradyarrhythmias or asystole are less common (20%). Evidence of coronary disease and healed myocardial infarction may be present, with acute infarction in only 20–25%, although this is population-dependent.

Investigations

Coronary angiography and exercise testing or perfusion imaging will together quantify the amount of coronary disease and whether inducible ischaemia is present. Holter monitoring and electrophysiological testing have a limited role in evaluating the presence of underlying arrhythmias, and their response to drug treatment.

Treatment

Revascularization may be required for patients with severe coronary disease, particularly if inducible ischaemia is present. A few patients may be candidates for surgical or catheter ablation of an arrhythmic focus. Anti-arrhythmic drug treatment in general is disappointing, due to the significant risk of arrhythmia recurrence. Defibrillator therapy is associated with a low risk of sudden cardiac death during follow-up; its use world-wide is increasing because of the limitations of drug therapy.

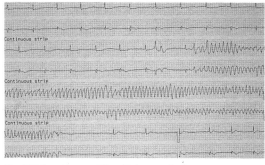

Fig. 149 Spontaneous VF on Holter monitoring.

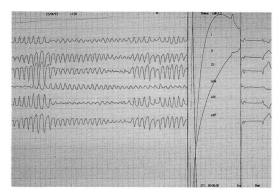

Fig. 150 ICD detects VF and delivers shock, restoring sinus rhythm.

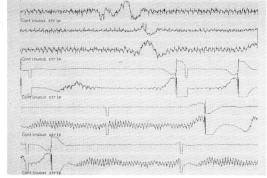

Fig. 151 Multiple shocks for VF delivered by ICD.

1–3% of attendances to casualty departments and 3–6% of hospital admissions are for syncope defined as a transient sudden loss of consciousness secondary to inadequate cerebral perfusion.

Aetiology

Simple fainting (vasovagal syncope) is the most common cause.

Arrhythmias should be considered in all patients. Bradyarrhythmias (Stokes–Adams attack) or tachyarrhythmias (e.g. ventricular tachycardia) may present with syncope.

Postural hypotension. Often due to drug therapy in the elderly, e.g. diuretics and vasodilators, or occasionally due to autonomic failure (Parkinson's disease, Shy–Drager syndrome etc.).

Obstructive lesions. Patients with aortic stenosis, hypertrophic cardiomyopathy and pulmonary hypertension may present with syncope.

Investigations

The key to management of these patients is a careful history. Evidence of high degree atrioventricular block or other conduction anomaly may be present on the resting ECG. Carotid sinus massage may reproduce symptoms and be associated with bradycardias. Ambulatory electrocardiography may reveal a specific cause such as ventricular tachycardia or paroxysmal atrioventricular block. In some patients with otherwise unexplained syncope, symptoms are reproduced by head up tilt, performed using a table designed for the purpose. In occasional individuals more sophisticated investigation such as electrophysiological testing may be necessary.

Management

Patients with syncope due to bradycardia detected during ambulatory electrocardiography or tilt testing, benefit from the insertion of a pacemaker. In other patients even after extensive investigations no specific cause is identified. The outlook for survival in these patients is excellent although morbidity may remain high.

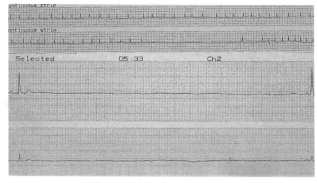

Fig. 152 Sinus node disease with prolonged pauses in patient with syncope needing pacemaker.

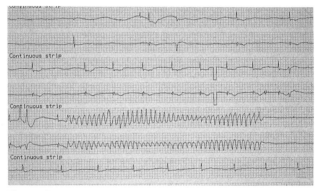

Fig. 153 Brady and tachyarrhythmias on Holter monitoring.

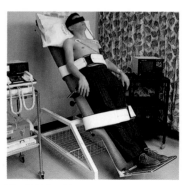

Fig. 154 Tilt table.

Pacemakers are highly cost-effective. In appropriate patients pacing cures symptoms and improves prognosis. More than 2 million pacemakers have now been implanted world-wide, but their use differs significantly between countries. In the mid 1980s use in sinoatrial disease in the US was 8 times that of the UK. Despite a decline in the US implantation rate of 25% in the late 1980s, rates are still in excess of those in Europe. Optimal implantation rates with present indications are probably around 300–400 units per million population per annum.

Indications

The main considerations are the improvement of symptoms and also prognosis.

Atrioventricular block. All patients with congenital complete heart block should probably be paced. Patients with acquired complete heart block (and probably those with 2nd degree AV block) should all receive a pacemaker whether symptomatic or not in order to improve prognosis.

Sinoatrial disease (sick sinus syndrome). These patients should receive a pacemaker if they have symptomatic bradycardia.

Presentation

Asymptomatic. Any patient found to have complete heart block should be referred for pacemaker implantation.

Symptomatic bradycardia. Patients with a slow pulse and dizzy spells, fatigue, dyspnoea, or congestive heart failure usually benefit from pacemaker implantation.

Stokes–Adams attacks. A patient with syncope and a history compatible with Stokes–Adams attack should be thoroughly investigated. Evidence of complete heart block is an absolute indication for the early implantation of a permanent pacemaker.

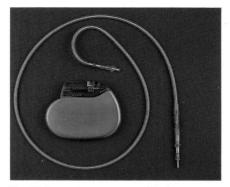

Fig. 155 Pacemaker generator and lead.

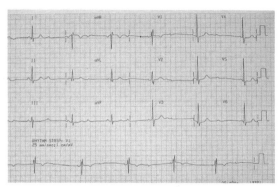

Fig. 156 Complete heart block. Atrial and ventricular activity dissociated.

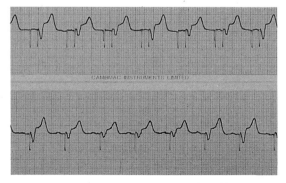

Fig. 157 ECG of dual chamber pacemaker pacing with appropriate sensed and paced atrial and ventricular activation.

Pacemakers (2)

Aetiology of conduction system disease

The majority of patients that need pacemakers have idiopathic degeneration of part of the cardiac conducting system. Coronary artery disease may also be present. In addition some patients with skeletal and heart muscle disease (e.g. dystrophia myotonica) may develop heart block. Kearns–Sayre syndrome is the rare combination of progressive external ophthalmoplegia, retinal pigmentary degeneration and progressive impairment of cardiac conduction. Other causes of heart block include infiltrative disease such as sarcoidosis, rheumatoid or amyloid, and infections such as Lyme disease.

Procedure

Relatively straightforward procedure under local anaesthetic; the pacemaker lead is advanced to the apex of the right ventricle (ventricular lead) or to the right atrial appendage (atrial lead), usually from the cephalic or subclavian vein and the pacemaker generator is then placed subcutaneously. The patient usually stays in hospital for approximately 24 h, although outpatient implantation is also successful.

Pacemaker types

An international code describes available pacemaker types. The most simple type of pacemaker currently used is the ventricular demand unit (VVI) which is relatively inexpensive, reliable and able to prevent major symptoms of syncope. VVI pacemakers do not provide coordinated atrial and ventricular contraction or increase the pacing rate on exercise. Rate responsive pacemakers (e.g. AAIR, VVIR etc.) have a sensor that increases the rate of discharge with physical activity. Dual chamber pacemakers (DDD) sense and pace both atrium and ventricle and provide atrioventricular coordination. Two pacing wires are required but they provide a more physiological replacement of the normal conducting system; the incidence of atrial fibrillation, stroke and left ventricular failure appear to be reduced when dual-chamber pacemakers are implanted in preference to VVI units in patients with sinus node disease.

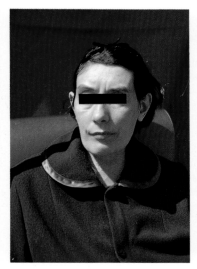

Fig. 158 Dystrophia myotonica.

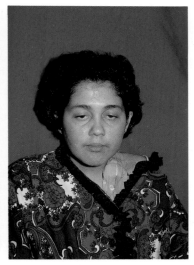

Fig. 159 Kearns–Sayre syndrome.

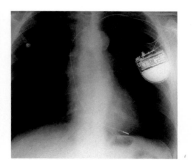

Fig. 160 VVI pacemaker (single lead).

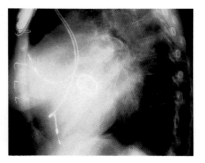

Fig. 161 DDD pacemaker (atrial and ventricular leads).

Pacemakers (3)

Complications of pacemaker implantation

If a patient presents with unexplained symptoms following pacemaker insertion the pacing centre responsible for that patient should be contacted.

Early complications

Lead displacement. May present with a recurrence of the initial symptoms if primary problem is loss of capture; if the problem is a failure to sense intrinsic cardiac activity then palpitations are more usual.

Early or late complications

Myoinhibition. Some patients complain of dizziness and occasionally syncope on arm movement due to myoinhibition—activity of the pectoral muscles is detected by the pacemaker leading to an inappropriate reduction of pacemaker discharge.

Infection develops in 1–2% and presents with pain over the pacemaker site. If the system is infected the entire unit must be removed. Infection usually presents in the first few weeks following implantation but occasionally much later.

Thrombosis. Oedema of the arm on the side of pacemaker insertion may occur (<1% of patients) and if severe may be improved by anticoagulation.

Pacemaker syndrome is a major disadvantage of VVI pacing. It is characterized by dizziness and heavy palpitations due to loss of properly timed atrial systole. Cure usually follows upgrade to a dual chamber system.

Late complications

Lead fracture or battery failure. Usually presents with recurrence of the initial symptoms.

Erosion. The generator or wire may erode through the overlying skin inevitably leading to infection. Early surgery is needed to limit infection.

Superior vena cava syndrome. Rarely patients develop stenosis of the superior vena cava with symptoms of upper body swelling and headache.

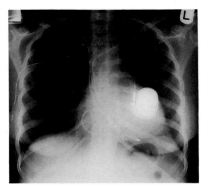

Fig. 162 Multiple pacemaker leads following many complications and procedures.

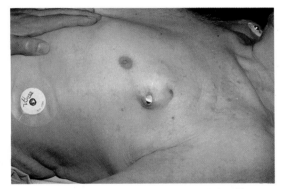

Fig. 163 Erosion of pacemaker generator through the skin.

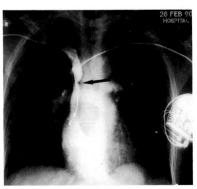

Fig. 164 SVC stenosis due to pacemaker lead.

The most common (30%) congenital heart abnormality detected in adult patients although 6% of congenital heart disease in children.

Classification

1. *Ostium secundum.* Most common type (70%). Located in the fossa ovalis, it occurs more commonly in females (ratio 3:1) and 20–30% have associated mitral valve prolapse.

2. *Sinus venosus* (15% of total). Occurs in upper portion of the interatrial septum and is often accompanied by partial anomalous pulmonary venous drainage.

3. *Ostium primum.* Sited in the lower septum and most commonly presents in childhood (often in Down syndrome) in association with other abnormalities.

Clinical picture

Adults present with fatigue, dyspnoea, palpitations and chest pain. The most characteristic signs are of wide fixed splitting of the second heart sound. A pulmonary flow murmur is usual, and with a large shunt a tricuspid flow murmur may be heard.

Investigations

Chest X-ray in uncomplicated cases shows a small aortic knuckle and pulmonary plethora. Later right sided chambers may become dilated.

Electrocardiography. Ostium secundum ASDs often have right bundle branch block which is usually incomplete (rSr' complex with QRS duration <0.10 s) and right axis deviation.

Echocardiography demonstrates the defect along with right ventricular volume overload and paradoxical septal motion.

Right heart catheterization. Demonstrates a *step-up* in oxygen saturation between the venae cavae and the right atrium allowing quantification of the shunt.

Management

Operative closure is usually recommended in symptomatic patients if pulmonary to systemic blood flow ratio >1.5:1.

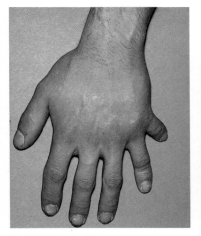

Fig. 165 Multiple digits may occur in patients with ASD.

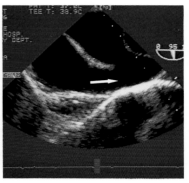

Fig. 166 Sinus venosus defect.

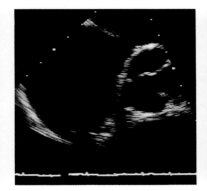

Fig. 167 Ostium secundum defect.

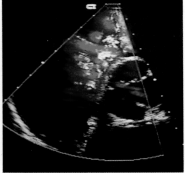

Fig. 168 Colour flow Doppler with flow across defect.

The most common congenital heart defect (30%) although the majority are detected before adulthood due to prominent physical signs. In addition to occurring as a congenital abnormality the defect may complicate acute myocardial infarction. The defect may occur anywhere along the ventricular septum but is most common in the membranous septum (70% of cases). It is seen in association with an ASD in Down syndrome.

Clinical picture

The presentation of VSD in adulthood is rare and usually follows the finding of a murmur or the development of complications. The classic murmur is harsh and pansystolic and sited at the lower left sternal edge. An accompanying thrill is usual. 5–10% have aortic regurgitation due to prolapse of a valve leaflet into the defect.

Investigation

Diagnosis is by echocardiography. Identification of small defects (Maladie de Roger) is facilitated by the use of colour flow Doppler. Chest X-ray appearances are non-specific but demonstrate pulmonary plethora due to increased pulmonary blood flow.

Management

Patients with small defects are managed expectantly with a greater than 30% chance of spontaneous closure in young patients. Large defects with a ratio of pulmonary-to-systemic flow >2:1 and right ventricular overload need surgical closure. Patients are at risk of endocarditis and should receive advice about antibiotics.

Fallot's tetralogy

Most common form of cyanotic congenital heart disease. Consists of pulmonary stenosis or atresia, ventricular septal defect, dextroposition of the aorta overriding the septal defect and right ventricular hypertrophy. Survival into adulthood is now common although patients remain at risk of a range of complications.

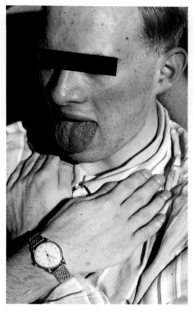

Fig. 169 Patient with Fallot's tetralogy.

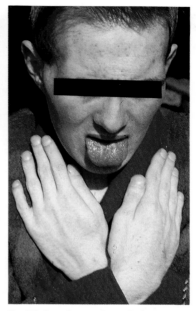

Fig. 170 Complete repair results in disappearance of cyanosis.

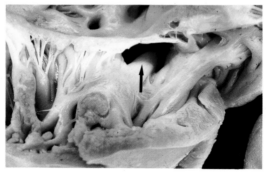

Fig. 171 VSD in Fallot's tetralogy

Pulmonary stenosis

10–12% of congenital heart disease. Acquired PS is unusual but may occur in rheumatic heart disease, following trauma and rarely due to the carcinoid syndrome (tricuspid stenosis with regurgitation is more common). Pulmonary stenosis may be part of the Noonan syndrome.

Clinical picture

Usually asymptomatic but may present with dyspnoea, easy fatiguability and occasionally chest pain and syncope on exertion. The key physical finding is of a systolic murmur at the upper left sternal edge. An ejection click is often present and the second heart sound is soft and delayed. There is usually a thrill in the same area.

Investigation

Chest X-ray. The pulmonary artery is dilated (post stenotic dilatation) and pulmonary vascular markings diminished with severe pulmonary stenosis. The right ventricle may be enlarged and occasionally is markedly so.

Electrocardiography demonstrates right axis deviation, right bundle branch block and evidence of right ventricular hypertrophy.

Echocardiography. Provides the diagnosis with Doppler allowing estimation of the transvalvular gradient and hence quantification of severity.

Management

Asymptomatic patients with mild to moderate stenosis do not need treatment and as the valve lesion is non progressive are unlikely to do so. Patients with moderate or severe stenosis (gradient >60 mmHg) and symptoms or with evidence of right ventricular dysfunction usually need treatment. This is now most efficiently carried out using transvenous balloon valvuloplasty.

Peripheral pulmonic stenosis

Some patients have supravalvular pulmonary stenosis which may consist of multiple narrowings of primary and more peripheral branches of the pulmonary arteries. This is often seen as part of the rubella syndrome.

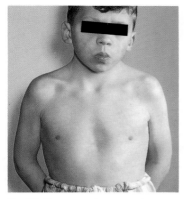

Fig. **172** Noonan syndrome.

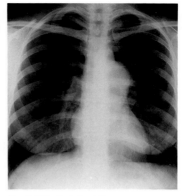

Fig. **173** Typical chest X-ray appearance.

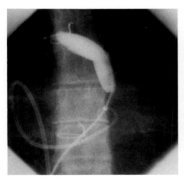

Fig. **174** Pulmonary balloon valvuloplasty.

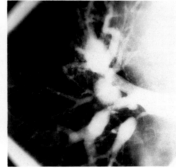

Fig. **175** Angiogram of peripheral pulmonic stenoses.

Coarctation of the aorta is due to a localized shelf-like thickening of the aortic lumen usually opposite the ligamentum arteriosum. In adults post-ductal coarctation is usual and males are affected twice as commonly as females. There is an association with Turner syndrome.

Clinical picture

Most adults with coarctation are asymptomatic but may have headache, claudication or fatigue. In women it may present with recurrent miscarriages. Coarctation is usually detected on routine examination with hypertension and diminished femoral pulses. Signs of a bicuspid aortic valve may be present (30%). A murmur is often present over the back due to collateral flow.

Investigations

Electrocardiogram. Evidence of LVH is often present.

Chest X-ray. Left ventricular enlargement is possible and notching on the lower posterior border of the third to eighth ribs is common. Pre- and post-stenotic dilatation of the aorta around the site of the narrowing may be seen.

Echocardiography is usually not definitive, but MRI may show the narrowed aortic segment.

Aortography. Identifies the site of obstruction, demonstrates the extent of collateral filling and also allows measurement of the pressure gradient.

Management

Mean life expectancy without treatment is 35 years. Death is usually due to complications of hypertension especially cerebrovascular disease (subarachnoid haemorrhage common due to the increased incidence of berry aneurysms), left ventricular failure or aortic dissection. Improvement in prognosis is achieved with surgery although hypertension usually remains postoperatively. In one study 70% of patients were hypertensive 30 years following surgery.

Treatment

Surgery remains the treatment of choice but long-term follow-up is essential.

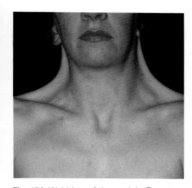

Fig. 176 Webbing of the neck in Turner syndrome.

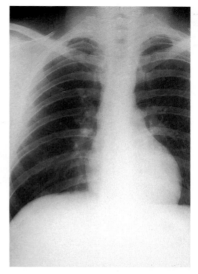

Fig. 177 Typical chest X-ray.

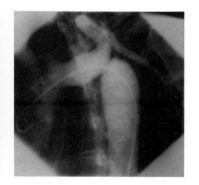

Fig. 178 Aortogram.

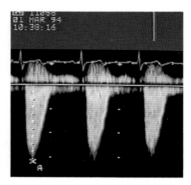

Fig. 179 Echo Doppler of coarctation with gradient of 40 mmHg.

Patent ductus arteriosus

Definition

Persistent arterial channel connecting aortic isthmus to the left pulmonary artery now seen rarely in adults.

Presentation

The anomaly is usually asymptomatic but there is a risk of developing heart failure, shunt reversal with development of Eisenmenger syndrome and bacterial endarteritis each of which may bring the condition to light.

Diagnosis

Continuous (machinery) murmur is of maximal intensity in the 2nd left intercostal interspace and may be the first clue to the problem.

Chest X-ray may show cardiac enlargement and pulmonary plethora. Calcification of the ductus may lead to a characteristic appearance in older patients.

Management

Ligation of the duct in childhood or resection in adults are curative if carried out prior to a rise in pulmonary artery pressure. Indicated in all patients to reduce the risk of complications.

Sinus of Valsalva fistula

Rare but the second most common cause of a continuous murmur in adult patients. Sinus aneurysms are either congenital or can occur secondary to infective endocarditis. Rupture usually occurs into the right ventricle and is associated with acute chest pain and possibly acute heart failure. The murmur is heard best in the second right intercostal space in most cases. Colour flow Doppler is diagnostic and the lesion can also be demonstrated by aortography. Surgical closure reduces the risk of ventricular dysfunction, infective endocarditis, septic pulmonary embolism and shunt reversal.

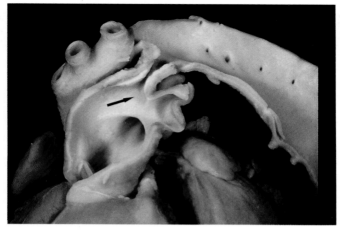

Fig. 180 Patent ductus arteriosus.

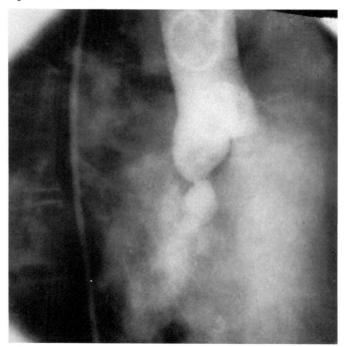

Fig. 181 Aortogram of sinus of Valsalva fistula showing flow between the right coronary sinus and the right ventricle.

Eisenmenger complex refers to a ventricular septal defect with pulmonary hypertension and right to left shunting of blood through the defect leading to systemic desaturation. Eisenmenger syndrome occurs following reversal of any left to right shunt (usually a VSD, PDA or atrioventricular septal defect and occasionally an ostium secundum ASD) following the development of pulmonary hypertension. Pulmonary hypertension develops due to thickening of the walls of the pulmonary arterial bed, the precise mechanisms of which are not established.

Clinical picture

Associated with symptoms of dyspnoea, easy fatiguability and haemoptysis. Cyanosis and clubbing are present. The unusual appearance of differential cyanosis with blue clubbed toes and pink lips and fingers occurs following shunt reversal through a PDA. Chest X-ray appearances may be bizarre with a very prominent pulmonary trunk and pulmonary arteries with peripheral oligaemia (*tree in winter*); evidence of right ventricular enlargement is often present.

Management

Individuals with cyanotic congenital heart disease including Eisenmenger syndrome commonly survive into adulthood. These patients have a number of special problems needing careful management. These include polycythaemia (need regular venesection), gout (prophylactic allopurinol often indicated), contraceptive advice (pregnancy usually poorly tolerated) and endocarditis. They often benefit from follow-up in a specialist clinic. Overall life expectancy is shortened. Selected patients may be candidates for heart-lung transplantation.

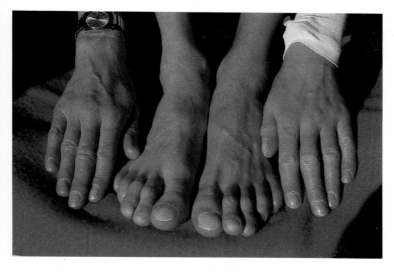

Fig. 182 Differential cyanosis and clubbing in patient with Eisenmenger PDA.

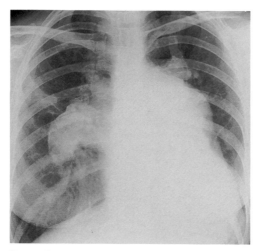

Fig. 183 Chest X-ray of Eisenmenger syndrome (ASD).

Thoracic aortic aneurysms

Aneurysms of the thoracic aorta are relatively uncommon. There are a number of causes:

Arteriosclerosis is the most common cause and may develop in any part of the thoracic aorta. The entire aorta may be ectatic and usually there is widespread arteriosclerosis elsewhere. The aneurysm itself is usually fusiform.

Cystic medial necrosis may result in annuloaortic ectasia and is a common component of Marfan syndrome and Ehlers–Danlos syndrome. Aortic dissection, rupture or regurgitation may develop. Annuloaortic ectasia is present in 5–10% of patients requiring aortic valve replacement.

Syphilis. Aneurysms develop in 5–10% patients with syphilitic aortitis. Patients develop a destructive aortitis which involves both the ascending aorta and the arch. Aortic regurgitation commonly develops due to involvement of the aortic valve cusps and angina may occur due to coronary ostial stenosis. Aneurysms may become huge and erode the sternum and ribs. On chest X-ray calcification in usually present in the aortic wall.

Management

Most patients are asymptomatic and come to light following a routine chest X-ray. Prophylactic surgical replacement is often needed in patients with large aneurysms but may carry significant risks.

Aortitis

Inflammation of the wall of the aorta is termed aortitis. Syphilis is a well recognized cause but is now uncommon. Other causes include ankylosing spondylitis, Reiter syndrome, ulcerative colitis and Takayashu's arteritis.

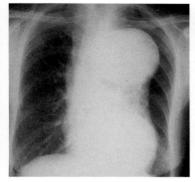

Fig. 184 Huge syphilitic aneurysm: chest X-ray.

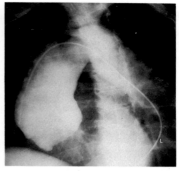

Fig. 185 An aortogram of the same aneurysm

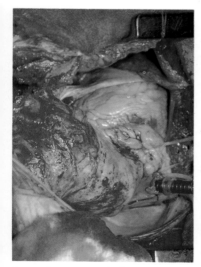

Fig. 186 The aneurysm in Fig. 185: intraoperative.

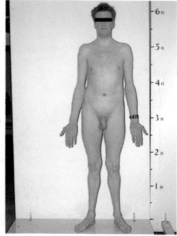

Fig. 187 Marfan syndrome.

Aortic intimal tear followed by tracking of blood into the aortic media. The usual site is the ascending aorta (type A) but other sites of origin are possible. Predisposing causes include hypertension (70–90% of patients have history of hypertension), Marfan syndrome, Ehlers–Danlos syndrome, bicuspid aortic valve and chest trauma. Males are affected more commonly than females (3:1) but dissection is described for example in pregnancy.

Presentation

Sudden onset of severe precordial or interscapular pain is characteristic. Blood pressure is often increased (in 50–70%) despite a shock-like state. An early diastolic murmur may be present. The crucial differential diagnosis is myocardial infarction.

Investigations

Chest X-ray. Abnormal in 80% with mediastinal widening and left pleural effusion being the most common abnormalities. However, the chest X-ray may be normal.

Electrocardiogram. Usually shows LVH resulting from predisposing hypertension but there are no specific changes. It helps to exclude other causes of chest pain, particularly myocardial infarction which may coexist with dissection (due to obstruction of the coronary ostia), although this is rare.

Definitive diagnosis. Transoesophageal echocardiography, Thoracic CT scanning, and MRI have high sensitivity in the detection of dissections but aortography may be required.

Management

Medical treatment with analgesia and beta-blockers is important. Immediate surgery is required in all patients with acute dissection of the ascending aorta. The ascending aorta is replaced with a prosthetic graft. Operative mortality remains however around 50%. Surgery for distal (type B) dissection is reserved for patients developing complications or Marfan syndrome.

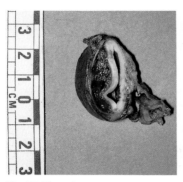

Fig. 188 Dissecting aneurysm (postmortem) with tracking of blood in the media and partial obliteration of the lumen.

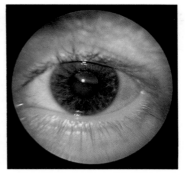

Fig. 189 Lens dislocation in the Marfan syndrome.

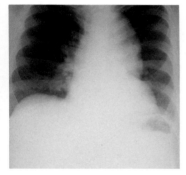

Fig. 190 Chest X-ray showing widened mediastinum.

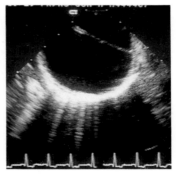

Fig. 191 Transoesophageal echo showing true and false lumens.

Complication of venous thrombosis usually arising in the deep veins of the legs. Some patients postoperatively are at particular risk (e.g. increased age, immobility, malignancy).

Clinical picture

Clinical diagnosis lacks sensitivity and specificity. Symptoms may include dyspnoea on exertion and at rest, pleuritic or central chest pain, haemoptysis and syncope. On examination the patient may be tachypnoeic, using accessory muscles, have a friction rub, a left parasternal heave and raised venous pressure or have no signs.

Investigations

Chest X-ray. Often normal and findings when present are non-specific, e.g. basal atelectasis. Most helpful in demonstrating another cause for the patient's presentation such as pneumothorax, pneumonia, pulmonary oedema etc.

Electrocardiography is often normal (>30%), or reveals a sinus tachycardia only. Changes such as $S_1Q_3T_3$ and RBBB are non-specific. The ECG may serve to exclude other possible causes of symptoms, e.g. myocardial infarction.

Lung scanning. Perfusion or ventilation-perfusion scanning is often useful as an initial diagnostic test. Mismatching of ventilation and perfusion with pulmonary embolism is a useful pointer to the diagnosis, but can be non-specific.

Pulmonary angiography. Reference for the diagnosis of pulmonary embolism shown as constant filling defects with a sharp cut off.

Management

Most patients require anticoagulation initially with heparin and subsequently warfarin. Patients with massive pulmonary embolism may be candidates for more aggressive therapy with thrombolytic agents or pulmonary embolectomy. Prevention of the passage of further clot from the deep venous system may be aided by the insertion of a caval filter.

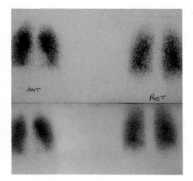

Fig. 192 Normal ventilation (upper) and perfusion (lower) scans.

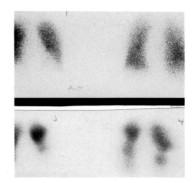

Fig. 193 Mismatch of ventilation and perfusion with multiple pulmonary emboli.

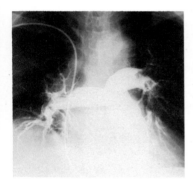

Fig. 194 Pulmonary angiogram showing filling defect and sharp cut off typical of pulmonary embolism.

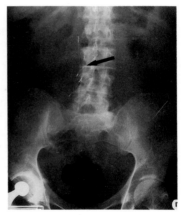

Fig. 195 Intracaval filter in situ.

Pulmonary hypertension is defined by a high pulmonary artery pressure and increased pulmonary vascular resistance. In many patients no cause is identified and the condition is termed primary pulmonary hypertension.

Clinical picture

The condition affects females more than males (ratio 5 : 1). Patients are usually young (age 15–40) and present with fatigue and exertional syncope, but chest pain or dyspnoea may be predominant. Patients may have evidence of a connective tissue disease with Raynaud's phenomenon and have a malar flush. On examination patients usually have peripheral but not central cyanosis when at rest. They may have an *a* wave visible in the venous pulse, a right ventricular heave and a loud pulmonary component of the second heart sound.

Investigations

Chest X-ray may show cardiomegaly with enlargement of the right-sided chambers, pulmonary artery enlargement with peripheral oligaemia (*pruning*), and a small aortic knuckle.

Echocardiography demonstrates a dilated right ventricle and paradoxical septal motion. Pulmonary artery pressure can be estimated.

Right heart catheter. Confirms diagnosis of pulmonary hypertension with a raised pulmonary artery pressure.

Pulmonary angiography. Usually required to exclude large vessel thromboembolism that may be helped with thrombo-endarterectomy.

Lung biopsy. Definitive test although similar changes can occur in Eisenmenger complex.

Management

A progressive downhill course is usual with a 10 year survival <25%. Most patients should receive anticoagulants and a trial of vasodilator therapy may be attempted with caution. Thrombo-endarterectomy or heart-lung transplantation should be considered.

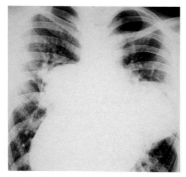

Fig. 196 Chest X-ray; primary pulmonary hypertension with massive proximal pulmonary arteries.

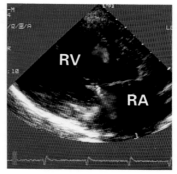

Fig. 197 Right ventricular enlargement on two-dimensional echocardiogram.

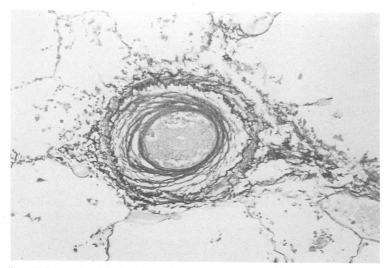

Fig. 198 Concentric thickening in a small pulmonary artery: lung biopsy histology.

75% of cardiac tumours are benign; the most common by far are myxomas, but lipomas, fibroelastomas and rhabdomyomas can also occur.

Atrial myxoma

Myxomas are thought to arise from primitive mesenchymal cells. 90% are atrial, four times more commonly on the left than the right. They are pedunculated and attached to the interatrial septum at the fossa ovalis. Patients may present at any age. In some the condition is familial. Patients may be asymptomatic, present with symptoms of mitral stenosis, with systemic embolism or constitutional symptoms such as lethargy, fevers etc. Findings on examination can be similar to those in mitral stenosis. Routine laboratory tests may be abnormal with normochromic normocytic anaemia, leucocytosis, raised ESR and gamma globulins. Chest X-ray appearances may resemble those of mitral stenosis though the left atrial appendage is not so prominent. The tumour may be calcified. Echocardiography is the investigation of choice. Angiography is no longer required but may produce dramatic images. Complete surgical resection is the treatment of choice

Malignant cardiac tumours

The most common are directly invasive from lung primaries or secondary deposits from elsewhere. Sarcomas are the most common primary cardiac tumours and present with heart failure, arrhythmias and effusions. The prognosis in these patients is extremely poor.

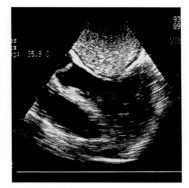

Fig. 199 Atrial myxoma on two-dimensional echo.

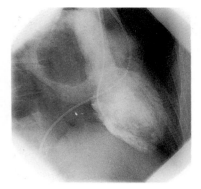

Fig. 200 Atrial myxoma on angiography shown as large filling defect after mitral reflux from LV angiogram.

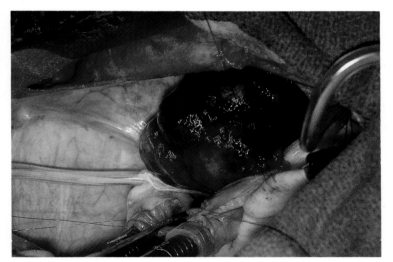

Fig. 201 Removal of atrial myxoma.

Index